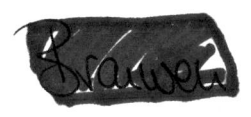

A Bite at a Time

From the Heart to the Mind,
Inspiration and Motivation for Weight Loss

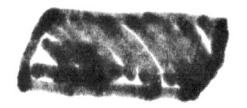

Wordclay
3750 Priority Way South Drive, Suite 114
Indianapolis, IN 46240
www.wordclay.com

© Copyright 2008 Morris C. Katzoff. All rights reserved.

No part of this book may be reproduced, stored in a retrieval system, or transmitted by any means without the written permission of the author.

First published by Wordclay on 1/7/2008.

Printed in the United States of America.

This book is printed on acid-free paper.

A Bite at a Time

From the Heart to the Mind,
Inspiration and Motivation for Weight Loss

Morris C. Katzoff

Dedication

This book is dedicated to my wife, Carol.

I often wondered silently how you could love this often crazy fat man and what you saw in me.

You are my inspiration, my motivation to succeed, and my strength. Your love, and faith in me, keeps me going.

Thank you for everything that you do for me. I know I say I love you often, but truly - I love you more than you will ever know.

Acknowledgments

I'd like to express my appreciation to the following people:

Norman Katzoff, (my Dad) who taught me about life and what it is to be a man. He has supported me in my endeavors. He has been an inspiration to me growing up, and he is my hero. His lessons have guided me; his common sense and advice has never steered me wrong. His wisdom continues to show me the way.

Mindy Tolchinsky, (my sister), who has always been there telling me "I can." She is always encouraging me at every turn and is probably my most enthusiastic supporter. He has helped me in so many ways, I couldn't even begin to express them all here because I'd run out of room.

John Van Epps, my best friend in life, my 'other' confidant, and my sounding board. He is always there for me whenever I need him - night or day. I don't know what I would do without him in my life. He is the definition of a true friend - more like a brother than simply a friend. I love him dearly. A successful copywriter (WritingDoneRite.com), he assisted with editing and marketing, and offered some suggestions and advice for this project.

Isabel Worden-Klym, author of *Old Friends and Ill-Starred Acquaintances*, who's hard, work am my editor has been invaluable to me. Her comments, insights and ideas have helped me throughout the writing of this book.

Foreword

One Bite at a Time is the seminal work of Morris Katzoff – my best friend and confidant – who for the twenty-plus years we've been friends – has fought a very personal battle against obesity.

Over the past two decades, I've seen both the joy and the heartache. The ecstasy of having the pounds melt away, seemingly effortlessly – and the pain of seeing the weight come back, like a ghost from the past, determined to continue its 'haunting.'

The ghosts are gone.

These past two years of Morris's journey has had a profound effect on me – not so much because I needed to lose weight (although I did), but because I've seen firsthand the results of a single-minded purpose, and how incredible those results can be.

I've learned much from his personal struggle – and his journey has inspired me to make some changes in my own life.

Morris has compiled an incredibly focused book of motivational and inspirational quotes, along with his personal commentary. Not a 'weight loss' guide, per se – no special diets, recipes, or 'how-to' regimen. Rather, it's a personal insight into the actual mindset that he's personally used to achieve his weight loss goals – and a tool *you* can use to make positive changes in your own life.

One Bite at a Time will be <u>your</u> inspiration to lead you to a better, more joyous, and more fulfilled life than you ever thought possible.

Enjoy!

John Van Epps

Introduction

A Bite at a Time is a book of motivational quotes with commentary. It does not profess to reveal any weight loss secrets, techniques, methodologies, recipes, or plans. It is not a "how to lose weight" book or a personal story of success. Instead it is interpretations based on Morris's observations and life experiences.

Morris Katzoff is a successful entrepreneur, a confidant to many, a weight loss / life coach and an inspiration to everyone with whom he comes into contact. His motivational messages will impact your everyday life because he understands the pain and torment of being overweight. He believes passionately about the manner in which words can influence the way people think and feel. Having lost over 200 pounds himself, he knows what it takes to reach inside and continue the struggle for another day.

Being on a weight-loss journey, we all need motivation and inspiration to stay on track. In compiling these quotations and expounding on them through his own personal experience and observations, Morris tries to make this book the ultimate tool for personal transformation.

With each quote he strives to bring new insight and meaning to the daily struggle of losing weight and the ongoing journey of reaching and maintaining our goals. You've seen these quotes in volumes of books; they are everywhere and are nothing new. But they might have meant nothing to you because they didn't relate to your personal experiences and struggle so they didn't 'speak' to you. Until now!

Each quote is accompanied by thought-provoking, profound and provocative commentary. Some are intended to be emotional; some are inspirational, while some are philosophical. Each reader will find that they interpret the quotations in a different manner; they will touch you and mean something distinctive to each of you depending on your own life experiences.

This book is perfect for anyone who has ever battled with their weight or is attempting to lose weight now. It will show you that you're not alone.

Finally, it is about hope and even though life contains many hardships, there are wins as well. Even though we suffer, there are also victories to celebrate.

A Bite at a Time will demonstrate to us all that we can lose weight as long as we never give up. We will survive and eventually find our way, by taking it "A Bite at a Time".

What Others Are Saying About This Book

Your book is really needed. It's important for a man's voice to be out there in the way that yours is. I'm meeting more and more men who need to hear that they are not alone and that there is hope.
Margaret Graham
CPCC,ACC
Professional Weight Loss Coach

"When you are struggling with weight loss, it is the big picture that haunts you. This is the pain of the overweight person stuck in the future. You believe you *will* be valuable when you are thin. You *will* be loved, and accepted. But you are already whole and already complete. Morris' book *A Bite at a Time* keeps you firmly grounded in that moment, in the journey. He provides simple direct quotations and reflections that zap you out of the future, where you really don't exist, into the present moment of your path. This is a valuable tool for staying on track. The truth is that this journey of weight loss is *A Bite at a Time!*"

Kelly LaCost
Easylife Coaching

"This author is intelligent and extremely thorough. I highly recommend *A Bite at a Time* and am grateful to the author for producing it. It really is a *masterpiece*. If you're currently trying to lose weight and <u>not</u> getting the results you want, I can tell you why right now. It's because you haven't read this book!!! ~ David G.

"I'm positively encouraged! I read A *Bite at a Time,* in one sitting, and was convinced this is what I needed to hear for a long time. I'm also certain that when people apply changing the way they think and use some of the principles Morris suggests in their day-to-day lives, they will experience a transforming effect on their life. ~ James H.

This is the best book I've read. I know without a doubt it will help me get what I really want from my weight loss plan.
~ Sue T.

This book really gets right to the heart of the matter -- and examines the basic reasons why we dieters often fail on our quest. Then, it gives simple, thought provoking takes on it, and enables us to change the way we think about our journey.
~ Nancy S.

This is a life changing book! I think I've finally found the real deal that is helping me to change the way I think, and feel about myself, my journey and how to make permanent lifelong healthy changes.
~Stephanie H.

"I read *A Bite at a Time* and it got me really excited about doing whatever it takes to make the necessary changes I need to make my diet a success. I began reading and re-reading it over and over, practicing many of the ideas in the book

faithfully. But not much changed for me. I began to think all this change your thinking stuff was completely *bogus.* But like the book said I stuck with it because something told me Morris had the right ideas here. After putting many of the ideas into action I realized there was a missing ingredient all along that kept me from my goals. It was - I wasn't practicing what I was reading, and when I started adding that missing ingredient, I was amazed at the results.
~ Scott J.

"I used to be really skeptical about anything that had to do with changing my attitude about things, positive thinking and the "just do it" mindset when it comes to succeeding at weight loss. While positive thinking has its advantages and has improved many people's outlook in life, rarely has any "normal" positive thinking, self help book changed my circumstances. Some helped a little and a few made me a more optimistic person. But none helped with my outlook when it came to my diet. So when I started reading this book, I remained extremely skeptical -- Finally, here's a book that tells it like it is -- and goes well beyond positive thinking. I've already seen positive changes in me and in my circumstances. It seems I'm not struggling as much these days with my weight and my life in general is getting better. *~ Paul T.*

One of the most insightful analyses written on how people like me who are trying to lose weight really think and how to change that thinking to bring about the changes we want from our weight loss program
~ Cindy D.

The best and most readable book on what it takes to make lasting, healthy choices every step of the way.
~Regina A.

A riveting narrative, based on the author's personal weight loss experiences that analyzes the basics and offers a shrewd insight into the over weight psyche.   *~ Wanda L.*

A Bite at a Time is crammed with nuggets of common sense. This book touches your heart strings. It is scholarly, reflective, motivating, encouraging and sympathtic   *~Leslie F.*

A reliable guide to an often painful subject; a book that gives its readers the mental ammunition to make sense of it all. This book manages to make us look honestly at ourselves which is a rare and welcome feat.
~ Cathy K.

Your messages have helped me keep focused on re-working my health habits. They keep me focused on my goal and quite frankly, self centered. I believe that has been a good portion of my problem that is, not putting myself first.
~ Peggy

I, too, struggle, and my decisions are poor at best on most everyday of my life. I weigh 300+ pounds and it is a nightmare to find clothes, fit in seats, and just function. Thank you for sharing your experiences, strength and hope.
~ Debra

I just had to let you know how much I enjoyed reading your book! It is thought provoking, encouraging and inspiring. Thanks so much!
~ *Barb*

Every time I REALLY followed a healthy eating program, it worked. But here is the rub; I either rewarded myself by going back to my old ways of felt deprived if I didn't.
 I also often fear failing again and again. That is why this book offers a very special kind of support. It shows we can succeed. When I think of the possibility of failure, it makes me weary. But I have also haven't had the kind of consistent encouragement that I have received from *A Bite at a Time*. So I am going with having a positive attitude and work towards success.
~ *Theresa A.*

I'm excited I found this book. I realize that weight loss is essentially a personal thing and we have to do it alone to a degree. But it helps to see there is someone who understands and can communicate to me the motivation I need to continue.
~*Frances C.*

I loved reading your book. It is fun for me to pursue the suggestions, and ideas. Also it keeps me out of the refrigerator.
~ *Monica B.*

For a long time I have been in the mind set that says "I can't lose weight". Now I have an "I can be successful" mind set.
~*Janice Y.*

A Bite at a Time has such great words of support and knowledge. I only hope that with time I can gain the wisdom needed to lose weight like you have.
~ *Darren Ii*

Thanks for your encouragement. I will now pass on to you the compliment given me by my toughest, crustiest journalism professor "You do good work."
~ *Pam R.*

It is obvious that what you write does indeed come from your heart. That is why *A Bite at a Time* is so special to so many of us. *A Bite at a Time* is incredible. I thought it was about time I told you that. You are so helpful to me and I am so grateful to have you (in a matter of speaking) in my life. Thank you once again for your inspiring book.
~ *Carla L.*

A Bite at a Time has had a great impact on me. I wanted you to know that I believe a lot of my new understanding of what goals are about and motivation (both health and diet) comes from reading your book. Thank You.. Thank You.. Thank You..
~ *Clair S.*

Your book, *A Bite at a Time,* has had a positive effect on me. I'm not eating as much. I'm developing greater awareness of food. My resolve is strengthening. Your wonderful insights are giving credence and reinforcement to my own thoughts. Instead of eating my meals in mindless obliteration, I am learning to make conscious choices. I have quit eating in front of my TV and or computer because of all your wonderful

suggestions. It really makes it hard to ignore what's going in my mouth. I'm a lot easier on myself too. *A Bite at a Time* has started me to get on track. I have decided that this time I am going to go slow and change my way of eating instead of dieting. Thanks again for making this possible for me.
~ Helen D.

My goal this year is not to diet but to eat healthy. I have been on so many diets and spent so much money on them that I am choosing to follow a new approach. Thank you for showing me the way.
~ *Carl R.*

First of all I wanted to say Thank You. I think *A Bite at a Time* is positively terrific. It is not only encouraging, but sincere and helpful. What more can I say, but thanks so much for your wonderful, understanding and supportive book.
~ Barbara M.

I am very grateful I found *A Bite at a Time*. As result I am starting to gain some control over my eating, and make wiser choices. Thanks again
~ *Samuel H.*

Thank you for the wonderful words of encouragement, understanding and caring. All the ups and downs, I face, the good days and bad together with all the helpful tips on what to try and what to avoid have given me courage and strength. With your help how can I not turn my failures into successes?
~Teresa A.

Thanks so much for all you do to keeping me on track. I know I couldn't have stuck with it for this long without *A Bite at a Time*.
~ *Love Wendy*

"Awesome read!!! It's a simple read -- took only me a few hours, but don't underestimate its simplicity. The author's depth of understanding and spirit really comes through."
~ *Linda V.*

My Story

As far back as I can remember I have been overweight. As an infant, I was the cute little baby with the chubby cheeks. As a toddler, I was chunky, but it was just baby fat and eventually I'd grow out of it. During my adolescent years I was wearing 'husky' size clothing and by the time I was a teenager I was out-and-out obese.

When I was young, I recollect sitting at a Weight Watchers meeting when a feeling of self-consciousness overcame me. It felt like my head was spinning and I became horrified as I realized that not only was I the youngest person in the room, I was also the largest person in the room. I couldn't believe my eyes. My heart was pounding. I began to sweat and tremble in disbelief. There I was in a room with people of all shapes and sizes, but I was definitely the fattest. Internally, I started feeling humiliated and as I sat looking around, I became more and more depressed. I mean, here I am at a meeting for fat people who want to lose weight and I'm the fattest one there! I never expected this to happen to me. The sensation was overwhelming and I felt very much alone in the crowded room. "The fattest person here" I thought over and over to myself. " This Couldn't be." Not me.

I stayed at the meeting that night only because I didn't want to get up and walk out. To do that, I would have had to pass almost everyone in the room. Although I felt extremely ashamed of myself, I continued to sit and listen even though what I really wanted to do was get up and run out of there. Yah, right, me run. That in itself would be a feat. I wanted to find somewhere to hide and cry my eyes out.

As I sat, people got up to share how they were doing that week with the group. One by one, they came up to the podium and told how well they did and what they did to stay on track. They were so inspiring. As I listened I recall thinking to myself "Yes, this is it." This is finally the program and diet that I needed to help me lose weight. After all, look at all these people. They're doing it so why can't I? For a moment I didn't even think back to all the other programs and diets on which I had previously been; the ones that failed me time and time again. I was excited and kept repeating to myself how I was going to do it this time so I would no longer have to be the heaviest person in the room wherever I went. I guess what I was really doing was trying to convince myself of all this, but in reality it felt more like an internal cry of hope than anything else. I suppose I would go so far as to call it a prayer. All the other diets and diet programs I ever tried had ended in disaster and all the time and money put into them was in vain. "This has to work," I thought. "Please make it work for me this time, God. Please!"

You would have thought the horror of this experience and the realization would have been enough to put an end to my overeating once and for all. The sad truth is, instead, that like so many times before, my hopes were soon dashed and turned into disappointment, despair and heartache. It really didn't matter what diet or weight loss program I was on because I'd tried them all and none of them seemed to work for me. Sure, I lost weight on the majority of these programs. In the end, I not only gained my weight back but weighed more than when I started!

I recall going to several doctors who tested me for thyroid problems, and had had me tested for all kinds of things to see if there was any reason medically why I was so heavy. I knew why I was heavy: I liked food and liked to eat. I didn't need a doctor to tell me that. My parents even sent me to a 'fat camp' in upper state New York one summer. I did great there and lost a considerable amount of weight but often wondered what was going to happen when I got back to the real world where food was abundant and all around me. I can still see the image of how proud my parents looked when they came to take me back home. I was decked out in all new clothes. I felt good about myself and also looked pretty good. After all these years, I really can't recollect how much weight I actually lost at camp, but I do remember that I was beaming from ear to ear. I was proud of myself; my confidence level was high, as was my self-esteem. My jubilation, though, was short-lived because it didn't take long after I got home to start gaining the weight back. All the temptations I wondered about while I was at the camp, were now calling my name, and, one by one, I surrendered to them. I don't think it was two months before all those nice new clothes I got at camp didn't fit me anymore. I eventually gained all the weight back that I lost, and then some. I was devastated and felt like a complete and utter failure. I let my parents down as well as myself. I found myself asking once again that all too familiar question, "Why me?" I lost faith in my higher power and inwardly cursed God. I wanted an answer as to why I had to be tormented and suffer so. What did I do in life to deserve this?

My teenage years were worse. By now I was miserable inside. I hated going outside, having to deal with all the crap I got from people. My self-esteem was at the lowest point that I had ever experienced. My spirit was crushed and I was one very lonely kid. Nobody wanted to hang around with the fat kid. I was an outcast and picked on daily, but never picked on for the team. I was always depressed and felt pretty hopeless when it came to any expectations of losing weight. I didn't want to go to school because I knew that I would be tormented there and ridiculed. More often than not, I got beaten up on the way home form school by several bullies.

But I kept trying. I never gave up. You've all heard the old saying, "If at first you don't succeed, try, and try again." I did just that: I kept trying. I have probably bought every diet book that has ever been published. I tried them all, but in the end, all I lost was my hard-earned money and my pride. Now don't get me wrong, most of the programs or diets that I tried worked for me. Some worked for a day, others worked a week and a few even worked a month or more. Every time something stopped me from succeeding. After a while, I either lost my motivation or just couldn't maintain my will power and enthusiasm anymore.

I often held conversations in my head about this. I'd do the best that I could to self-examine why or what it was that led me to fail once again. I'd ask rhetorically, "What's wrong with me?" "Why is it that these other programs work for everyone else, but I can't stay on one past a few months?" I would even ask God if I was being punished for something. "Why me?" I'd ask, "Why me?" I felt like an outcast and a freak. After all, I was different from all the other kids. They were normal. They weren't overweight. They dated, played sports, went out, hung around with friends, went to the prom and did all the things kids do. Not me. I was more times than not at home, alone, wallowing in my misery.

Looking back to those teenage years and going back even before my teens; I see that I always weighed two hundred fifty pounds. At least that is what my driver's license indicated, as did other documents. I was so ashamed of my actual weight, that whenever I filled out any sort of paperwork that asked for my weight, I automatically wrote in two hundred fifty pounds. One day, while rummaging through my desk, I came across my driver's licenses for the years 1982 and 1992. The reality I didn't want to face or admit to myself or anyone else was that I weighed closer to five hundred fifty pounds. As I grew older, I gained even more. Funny, but I didn't feel like I weighed so much. I certainly didn't see myself as some gigantic overweight fat slob. Additionally, there were lots of times I actually felt "normal."

That was until I glimpsed at a mirror or noticed my reflection as I passed by a window. Then it would hit me. That was me in the mirror, or that was my reflection. I immediately snapped back to myself and thought that that couldn't be me. I was disgusting; fat didn't even describe me. I was obese, huge, enormous, and mammoth! I loathed that image that looked back at me to the point that I broke down in tears. I thought, no wonder everyone picked on me. Why wouldn't people make fun of me? I looked like the circus fat man! No wonder that I was picked on and beaten up every day at school. If I was normal, I'd beat myself up too! One glimpse was all it took to be reminded of my size, and I thought, "And you wonder why people don't just leave you alone or constantly call you names? You really don't get why they torture you and humiliate you at every opportunity. Do you really think you don't deserve the glares, the pointing fingers and the laughter?"

No wonder that I have but a handful of friends. Some of the friends I did have saw me as the class clown or the jolly fat kid who made them all laugh. That was only so they wouldn't laugh at me. I never could "get the girl" for that matter. I didn't go out on dates and the prom was so far form my reality that I didn't even dream about that special night. Basically, I didn't experience any of the things that normal kids did. But my story isn't all that unusual, for many kids who grew up were fat. Many of you who are reading this story, can associate all too well with what I am relating to you. I know you've cried the tears, experienced the pain, the torment, the humiliation. You've suffered in ways people who have never been overweight will never know or understand. I'll wager that there were even times that you wished you could just crawl into a corner and die.

I had a "fat friend" named John. He was my best friend at the time. Together, we could be ourselves and not worry about the world and what people thought about us. We hung out a lot; we understood each other, although we never really talked much about our size. We were the type of "buds" that you had for life, or so I thought. One day I called his house to see if he wanted to get together. I spoke to his sister and immediately knew from her voice that something was wrong. She was older than John and explained that he had committed suicide. I hung up the phone in shock and disbelief. As the tears ran down my face, I understood for a fleeting moment that his pain had become too much. I also wished I were dead. Life was that tough then. It took every ounce of energy I had to get up and face the world. Then, I thought, John took the easy way out. He had abandoned me, and his family. I felt so alone; I could never bring myself to talk with his sister, mom or dad about John after that. I didn't go to his funeral or ever see any of the family again. I think of John every now and then, and wonder what kind of a man he would have been today. I wonder if he would have married and had children. I think, as hard as it was, life is still worth the struggle. I miss him.

My childhood and teenage years were literally a living hell. Most of my adult years weren't too much better, yet I never did anything about it. Every year, I recall saying to myself, "When I turn twenty, I will finally go on a diet and lose weight." That became twenty-five, then thirty, then thirty-five, and forty. Year after year, I made the resolution that this would be the year I would buckle down and lose weight. We all know what happens to resolutions and I was no different.

Today, I'm married which frankly is something I never dreamed would happen to me. I met a wonderful woman named Carol. Since my childhood was filled with ridicule and torment I really didn't want to risk bringing children into the world, fearing they might be fat like me and have to endure what I did. So I made a vow never to have children to myself and my creator. The thing I liked about Carol was she already had children. At the time we were married the children were young, today between them I have four wonderful grandchildren.

Everyone who meets Carol and I comments about the love they see in our eyes for each other even after all these years together. We were married in 1985. Carol is the best thing that has ever happened to me. I know much to my experiences good and bad that I have encountered throughout my life has formed me into the person I am today. Some of these experiences are painful, and cut deep into my memories - others take my mind to a wonderful place of peace, joy and tranquility. Some still take my breath away, like when I asked Carol to marry me - and she said "yes".

At the moment I am a successful entrepreneur. On the side I am a personal coach, mentor, and motivator to many people. I enjoy my life, although I still struggle with my weight. And for those ask and they often do I follow the Carbohydrate Addict's Life Span Program by Drs. Richard F. and Rachael F. Heller. To help keep me on my program I attend a fantastic weight loss support group every week called T.O.P.S. (Take Off Pounds Sensibly). By attending weekly meetings it keeps me accountable and loyal to my program especially considering there are weekly weigh-ins. Not to mention I have met many amazing people there some of which have become close personal friends.

I'm not perfect by any means. I do the best that I can, looking positively on life and the circumstances we face as much as I can. The life I had I wouldn't wish on anyone. What I had to endure growing up should have never happened. I try not to figure who's to blame. Was it me? Drs Heller a long time ago taught me it wasn't. Was it the mean spirited kids I went to school with or the bullies that would beat me up just because I was different? Was it the name calling and all the other outside forces that I constantly had to thwart off at every turn? You know it doesn't matter anymore where the blame lies. The fact is many of my childhood years still haunt me every now and then, like it was yesterday. Those deep seated wounds sometimes open up without warning or provocation and cause me great pain and anguish even to this day. Really it doesn't happen that often and when it does I get over it pretty quick. I use my positive inner voice to remind myself that those kids and mean spirited adults put me through doesn't matter anymore. The truth be told I've forgiven them a long time ago.

Don't get me wrong I am delighted and extremely thankful that the teasing, the name calling, taunting and the laughter are long behind me now.

All these experiences have made me the man I am today, and somehow along this journey we call life I discovered that I liked myself. The best part is that person who had been hidden by the many layers of fat is much more visible these days. I am strong, compassionate, caring and sympathetic. I am a survivor and a conqueror that has made peace.

To be honest, if I had it to do all over again, I doubt I'd change much if anything about my past. If it wasn't for my being obese, the many issues I faced, and the pain, along with the struggle. I recognize I wouldn't be the person I am today. I am an accumulation of my past so if I changed any of it, I know I wouldn't be the person I am today. It is my experiences past and present that allow me to forge on.

I'm looking for Stories

I'm looking for stories! I would love to hear from you for my next project entitled, *Dear Friends You're Not Alone* ™

Dear Friends You're Not Alone is about you. It's about me, it's about us. It is about what it feels like to be overweight; what it is like to walk in our shoes for a day or a specific instance. It pulls the façade off the "Jolly Fat Man" image with which we are associated. It deals with the pain we live with daily, both physically and mentally.

Dear Friends You're Not Alone is about the long journey of losing weight; it's about the torment of growing up fat. The struggle and the daily battle that only those of us who travel this road understand. It is detailed accounts of what we go through. It is about our battle to stay in control and what it takes to stay motivated and determined to achieve our weight loss goals. It is reflections of what we missed out on in life, or the things we could have done or been if it weren't for our size.

It's about the humiliation and ridicule we have endured and face all the time. It's about other people's ignorance and the many obstacles we must overcome just to survive without going mad or committing suicide. The book will be your stories of the perceptions people have of the so-called jolly fat man or woman, and how they see us. It is about being torn apart inside by the laughs, jeers and stares we get. It's about not being able to sit in a booth in a restaurant. The book will share the shame we feel when we overeat or binge and go off our diet. The self-hatred we experience; the fears we have about our health and the many emotions we suffer having to live in a thin person's world.

Dear Friends You're Not Alone is also about our determination not to give up. It is about real people and real experiences. It is the real results we have made in our lives to lose weight and the healthy and positive changes that we have accomplished.

Together we will learn about what it takes to stay on track, the methodologies we employ without all the hype from people trying to sell us on their diets programs or products. We will reveal what keeps us motivated, what we say to ourselves to stay inspired and or having the ability to develop and improve in spite of the continuous hurdles we have to endure every day. Most import together we will learn "You are not alone"

A Bite at a Time™

"I try to take one day at a time, but sometimes several days attack me at once."

~Ashleigh Brilliant

In addition to changing how we think to achieve permanent success we need to undertake a new approach of getting immediately back on track when we do falter.

"Take it a day at a Time" - We have all heard of this concept taught by most programs that are committed to dealing with addictions, whether it is alcohol, overeating or substance abuse. It is also a concept used in grief and other types of counseling. The reason it is so often quoted is that it is universally applicable to so many situations.

Haven't we all had days, weeks and maybe months like that! The problem with taking it a day at a time for someone who is trying to eat healthier and lose weight is that if you go off your program and internalize this way of thinking, you also give yourself permission to eat uncontrollably for the day. This only leads to feelings of guilt to the point that we become overwhelmed and often scared that we'll never get back on track.

We must learn to be kinder, gentler and more patient with ourselves and not let our emotions control us. When we do detour from our goals, we know it's only temporary. Granted, it is always unexpected and often at the most inopportune times. You may, for instance, be driving by a McDonalds like you have successfully done a hundred times, but for some unknown reason something triggers your desire for one and you are thrown into a sudden spiral and are out of control. When this happens, instead of taking it a day at time, allowing your self the luxury of continuing to eat out of control for the rest of the day, take it "A Bite at a Time" TM.

The concept of taking it "A Bite at a Time" is clearly far superior than taking it a day at a time. When you utilize the Bite at a Time method, you immediately get back on track by making the next piece of food you put in your mouth one that is healthy and part of your eating program. This is much better than continuing to be out of control for an entire day pigging out on food. This offers us a fuller and, most important, a healthier, less stressful life. It takes us back to our goals and dreams without delay, devoid of all the drama and anxiety we bring upon ourselves.

Positive Thinking

"Being positive or negative are habits of thoughts that have a very strong influence on life."

~Remez Sasson

You've heard positive thinking and the way you think about yourself, your diet, your health and your eating plan to lose weight influences how and when you will achieve your goals. It manipulates how you stay motivated and how we follow through. It is the whole premise of *A Bite at a Time* and what it takes to complete our journey.

Frankly, there is too much emphasis placed on diets. Permanent weight loss is not all about food. Think about it, there are literally hundreds of books written that all profess to have the ultimate answer on how to lose weight, yet, interestingly enough, they are all different. If you were to boil them down to their core elements, they all agree that you need to eat less and exercise more to lose weight. One ingredient that seems to be missing from the majority of these books, although a few comment on but most completely fail to acknowledge is how our thinking literally affects our overall success or failure when attempting to lose weight. The way we think influences how we stay motivated, and dictates our commitment levels, and our follow through.

There is too much attention and emphasis written on how to lose weight when it is a known truth that the majority of us who have traveled this often arduous and difficult journey already know how to lose weight. After all, we have successfully done it many times over, only to gain it all back.

For some we have even reached our goal weight. Many of us call this syndrome yo-yo dieting. The very first thing then that we need to do for ourselves is to admit we can lose weight because we've done it before. That means there is no medical reason that we are not losing. We simply need to stop using this excuse and get away from telling ourselves that we can't lose weight. How can we continue down this road, when we know in our hearts that we have already proven we can do it?

This means it is time to give some serious thought as to the why's, and what barriers are keeping us from reaching our destination. What is it exactly that is preventing us from losing or keeping our weight off permanently?

Without getting technical or delving into the psychology of a fat person, the reality is that it all boils down to gaining control over our negative self-destructive self-talk. In essence, that is the missing link in the vast majority of diets and eating programs.

Many of us who have been struggling with weight already understand this concept, but for some reason just don't accept it as reality or make positive thinking part of our daily routines. The good news is that you can choose to lose, simply by eliminating the negative self-talk and destructive thinking right now, in addition to how you think about your past failures. By taking responsibility for your actions you can turn this cycle around almost immediately. There is no truth that if you diet and lose weight, you will only gain it back. You can stop this sequence once and for all.

For some there may be generics involved and in a few cases legitimate medical reasons for our weight, but typically it is our own repeated internalized negative messages that are our stumbling block and our nemesis.

Change your thinking and you change your results. You have to do this because food is everywhere we turn. It is always going to be there, calling our name and tempting us. We are literally bombarded with messages about food everywhere we go and every time we turn on a television. There is no getting around them. As a society, we are much too obsessed with food. Once you recognize that it is your own negative thinking that is keeping you from not only achieving your goals but making them permanent, you will soon find that your weight loss journey will become much easier.

Adopt a no more excuses approach to weight loss along with a no more stinking thinking position and you will experience unbelievable changes in your program. Negative, self-destructive thinking only destroys your hopes, dreams and ability to be successful; not only on your weight loss plan, but in everything you do in life. Can you guess how many times people like Thomas A. Edison were told something wouldn't work or couldn't be done? How about some of our most successful entertainers, athletes and entrepreneurs? How many times do you think someone told them that they couldn't or wouldn't do something, or amount to anything or achieve their goals? Likewise you have to stop sending yourself these same negative self-defeating messages. There is no such word as 'can't' because if you want something bad enough and are willing to make changes, you will accomplish them.

The only thing keeping us fat if we are doing our best to follow a diet or a healthy eating plan is the way we think and how we treat ourselves. Our thoughts do control our actions, so decide now that you 'can' and suddenly you will slowly start seeing that you become a doer instead of a wisher or a hoper.

When you accomplish this, you will feel better about yourself. Before you know it, that negative self-talk will take a back seat in your life, and positive thinking will dominate your actions, and increase the longevity of your success. The more you practice changing your thinking, not only does it become easier but is also formulates deeper roots in your mind that will increase your self-confidence and outlook on every thing you do.

It is actually amazing what we can do with our minds and how we can use positive self-talk to inspire ourselves right to that finish line. We don't have to give up or give in, or conform to what people tell us what can or can't be accomplished or what we personally can achieve.

Many people who believe what we put out into the universe, we get back. It is known as the Law of Attraction. The more you practice this concept, the more positive results you will experience in your program. This will allow you the opportunity to focus more clearly on you and become your personal best. In fact, the more you achieve, the more compelled you are to continue making changes. There is nothing like results to catapult your enthusiasm into high gear. You will become your most fervent supporter even in times when there are obstacles that will want to prevent you from becoming anything you want to accomplish, whether it is weight loss or anything else in your life.

One thing you are going to have to do in regard to being more positive is to surround yourself with optimistic, upbeat people and remove all negative influences and people from your life. That may be a lot to ask but if anyone is worth it, you are. It may be a difficult task to demand from you; however, in the end you will see the value and how this one action alone will add to changing your negative thinking and your weight loss success. Your main concern right now has to be you, not other people, or how and what they think. By eliminating negativity in all its various forms it will do nothing but improve your health, appearance , and how you feel about life and the way you look at the world. With this dedication, determination, and fortitude, nothing can or will stop you. Accept this as fact and it will become your new reality to the point even you will be in awe of your accomplishments and how far you can go altering your damaging thinking and move beyond being fat to fit.

None of us wants to be fat; none of us would choose this lifestyle if asked. I doubt that any of us would accept our size or the numerous limitations it puts on us if give the choice. Especially if we knew beforehand what we know now. Our burden is just too immense. Many of us silently wonder how we can endure another day because our struggle is so overwhelming sometimes.

You are not doomed as long as you create this one very necessary change in your attitude and what self-talk you use. Why pay thousands of dollars like many people have for weight loss counseling in search of the Holy Grail of what the answer is to changing their past behaviors so they can put an end to failing at the weight loss efforts. Weight loss is complicated at best, because for many of us there are psychological as well as physiological components to being overweight, fat or obese. Unfortunately for many of us, this is just another excuse or perceived reality.

Change for many of us is very uncomfortable. If we can just get out of our comfort zones long enough and "think about what we were thinking," we can gradually change any negative thinking, thoughts, emotions, or ideas that enter our minds . We can start seeing different results that will last a lifetime.

Snake Oil Salesmen

" If you can't dazzle them with brilliance, baffle them with bull."
~ W.C. Fields

In today's society it seems that the onslaught of diet commercials is everywhere. Their message is fueled by a thirty-five million dollar industry trying to part you from your hard earned money. "Eat More Weigh Less," "Twenty Pounds in Three Weeks," "Ten Pounds in Ten Days," "Be Thinner, Be a Winner," "Guaranteed Weight Loss." The list goes on and on. For the most part they promise some sort of breakthrough discovery that will have you losing weight fast, and easily without hardly any effort at all.

Well it's all a bunch of bull. There is no magic pill or supplement, miraculous formula or fad diet that is quick, easy and permanent. If there was we would have known about it by now. Heck they wouldn't even need to advertise it on TV. Losing weight takes effort and commitment; there is no way around it. While some products may work temporarily and bring results, they aren't the best way in the world to lose weight.

Truth be told, losing weight is as simple as it is difficult. To lose weight you need to eat less calories than you burn. You also need to increase your activity level and decrease the amount of calories you consume.

Americans are obsessed with these fad diets. They are popular because they have a few things in common. They promise a quick fix and fast results, they are somewhat easy to follow and claim unbelievable results. Most promote themselves as the best approach to losing weight. I say unbelievable because, as dieters, if we used our logic when we see one of these so called amazing diets we would remember we've been there and done that. We've tried similar programs and they've failed. Not only did they fail, most likely you gained weight after going off it.

Unfortunately they also have another thing in common: they don't promote sound weight loss and they only work short term if they work at all. They also rarely if ever promote any type of exercise. They tell you that you can lose weight in your sleep or you don't need to exercise on their program. In addition most if not all are nutritionally inadequate.

Bottom line is this: the best weight loss program out there is one that promotes eating less, physical activity, is high in vegetables, fruits, complex carbohydrates, and low-fat dairy products. Some promote low-Carbohydrate intake and protein consumption and finally they are convenient and inexpensive.

Now wouldn't it be great if there was that magic pill out there for shedding those hard to lose extra pounds? Most people aren't fooled by these fad diets and realize there is no quick-fix. They know that to lose weight and maintain it, it is going to require that you make many lifestyle changes. It's a difficult task and takes long term determination. It's important that you not be fooled by them and waste your hard earned money anymore.

Long term weight loss is a life-long commitment. It takes the willingness to change not only how you eat, what you eat and to get moving but your thought processes as well. That is what "A Bite at a Time" encourages you to do.

You don't need to look for unhealthy fad diets and quick weight loss. You need to take losing weight at a slow and steady pace. There is nothing new about losing weight. Living in a "Time Challenged" age we want everything now. While that's great for some things, it is not great when it comes to losing weight. Overall, there is nothing better than taking it slow, two-three pounds a week. Getting people to be patient with themselves and to take it slow, however, is difficult and challenging at best.

How serious are you about meeting your weight loss goals? If you can be patient, lose weight smartly, slowly and commit to the long-term. Be realistic about your goals and do whatever it takes to reach them. Far too many people desire results but aren't willing to put forth the effort to reach them. So many people want so much not only from a weight loss plan but they want to achieve financial freedom as well. The problem is the level of commitment. We give up too soon, for many people stop within sight of their goals.

We have to realize that there is no magic wand pill or diet, so you are just going to have to get serious and do whatever it takes, as long as it takes, without faltering. You have to be willing to invest time, lots of effort and hard work in your future health and well being. You have to give up the excuses. Stop feeling you should do more and do just do it. Once you have made up your mind to lose weight, go for it with a positive attitude.

Hope

"Hope is always available to us. When we feel defeated, we need only take a deep breath and say, "Yes," and hope will reappear."

~*Monroe Forester*

When we are working very hard and sticking to our weight loss plan, only to step on that scale and see a gain, it is tempting to throw up our hands and give up. There is no doubt in your mind that you did everything correctly; you didn't cheat once and made a real, honest effort. You gave your program your all only to see everything you worked so hard to achieve was for nothing. You look in shock at the scale feeling frustrated, discouraged, disappointed and angry, wondering why you even bother any more.

Feelings of self doubt and hopelessness slowly steal your desire to stay on your plan, and all your enthusiasm begins disappearing as you gaze at that scale in total disbelief. The temptation of just calling it quits right there and then twirl through your head in utter bewilderment.

The reality is that we have all been there before at one time or another. It's painful and cuts deep into our sense of self worth and resolve to go on. It is these moments when we feel crushed that we must stop, take a deep breath, clear our thoughts and not lose sight of what we have accomplished thus far. We must keep in mind the goals we have set for ourselves, not allowing a number on a scale to shape the rest of our journey. If you do, something magical will happen.

Every Journey Has to Start Somewhere

"Though no one can go back and make a brand new start, anyone can start from now and make a brand new ending."
~ Carl Bard

Right now is an opportunity to get started towards reaching your goal. Nothing is stopping you and nothing is standing in your way except maybe you.

You need to get out of your own way and eliminate whatever obstacles you're placing in your path. Normally these obstacles manifest themselves in the form of excuses as to why you can't stick to your diet, why you can't lose weight, why you have no motivation, etc. It's easy to never take the first step on the road to losing weight as long as you have an excuse. It's simple to justify every move in your head, but come on, you know better. Is it laziness? Maybe it's your lack of belief in yourself and your ability to stick to your program. Or is it your past failures that are holding you back?

If this is the case, it isn't logical that your future happiness and ability to achieve your weight loss goal should revolve around your past. Now is the time you have to stop measuring your self worth and your future happiness on your past performances.

Lets start by polishing your self esteem and confidence today and wipe your mind clean of the "It's". It's too hard, it takes too long, it's impossible for me to lose weight, my weight is going to come back, it takes too much will power, it's not enough food, it's too strenuous for me to exercise, it's useless keeping a food log, it's hard to keep track of my calorie intake every day. It's it's, it's …. "It's" are nothing more than another name for excuses.

Yes, excuse, my friend and everyone has one. You have to prevent your inner voice from telling you anything other than you're going to lose weight this time around. You're not a weak-willed loser. We all have within us the power to make changes and begin a new journey in a new direction at anytime we desire if we want it bad enough.

Being overweight does not have to be your destiny. It isn't predetermined prophecy; you have the willpower and determination to succeed at losing weight in spite of what many people believe. Every one of us who is overweight knows we have will power in ways most people who don't battle with a weight problem will never comprehend. In addition, willpower is much more than our ability to stick to a diet or to push food away once we're feeling full.
It is our strength of character and our moral character too; it is our capacity to face the day in a thin man's world. We know it can be pretty scary out there sometimes, having to deal with the prejudices of people and their constant assumptions about those of us who need to lose weight. It's sickening because we have more perseverance than most people do. We continue to fight to lose weight everyday and don't give up, yet we have to endure people's torment and discrimination.

So you have willpower and much more of it than most people. Seriously think about this for a moment. How many people out there could face what we do and keep going day after day? Many people would cave in to the pressure society places on us and crawl into a hole and never come out. How many people would keep at something, fail at it, then brush themselves off and start over again and again? We do, that's who.

It is time to start convincing yourself you have the power or willpower if you want it to achieve. You're not a failure, you have self respect, you have self control, you are not worthless, and you're not a loser or any person's definition of you. Your definition of you is what you make it. So start today, by visualizing the you that you want to become. Forget all the "It's." Wipe out all the excuses that you've tabulated in your head and use whenever you're faced with a difficult day or obstacle on your program. Retrain your inner voice because it is your thinking that needs to be rewritten, reprogrammed, and replayed often in a more caring, positive and constructive manner.

When an "it's" or an excuse finds its way in your mind, rewrite it. If you start thinking it's too difficult to stay on my diet, rewrite that thought. Reprogram your thinking to "Today I will stay on my diet," then replay that thought over and over in your mind until that little negative voice gets further and further away until you can no longer hear it or recognize what it is saying. If your inner voice tells you that you're a loser, rewrite that thought, reprogram your thinking to "I am a winner, I am doing this and I'm darn proud of myself." If you find yourself thinking I can't, rewrite that thought; reprogram your thinking to "I can."

All you have to do is take that first step and get started on this journey of rewriting your thinking. You don't need anyone else's opinion, pat on the back, reinforcement or recognition. You can do this alone and make your positive self-persevering inner voice your constant companion and supporter that will always be there to cheer you on.

Our Little Inner Voice

Dieting can be downright discouraging at times. Especially when you have worked hard for days, weeks or months, and all of sudden something goes wrong and you start in on a bingeing frenzy. Once started, your little inner voice starts talking to you, telling you what a failure you are and asks lots of negative non-productive questions like "what's the use? All this hard work and for what, now I'm off my diet again? It's too hard to stay on this diet, etc." You start beating yourself up and begin the process of doing everything and anything to keep you from attaining your goals.

The frenzy continues and before you know it you're completely off your program and have little or no control left. Your motivation to get started again is nonexistent. It is just about this time that the self-inflicted mental abuse starts; your little inner voice tells you what a failure you are. Then your little inner voice proceeds to become meaner and more hateful toward yourself than anyone has ever been to you. The cycle goes on for some time and you become depressed and even more discouraged and at some point lose all hope of ever getting back on your diet.

Sometimes that little inner voice (the helpful more pragmatic voice) kicks in and tells us we have to get back to our diet. It tells us we want to get back, we need to get back. It tells us we'll feel better if we do and of course we agree.

But that little inner voice (the one that discourages us), like the devils of good and evil, one on each shoulder, starts in again. What's the use, go eat that box of cookies, you deserve it.

It's too hard to diet, besides you've failed for years. You're a failure; you're a pig, it's too late, you blew it.

We have to train our little inner voice (the helpful more pragmatic voice) to speak up more often and louder. We need to train it to shout at us so it can be heard over all that negative talk.

When the time comes you hit a bump in the road of your dieting journey (and it will), you need to stop that little inner voice (the one that discourages us). You need to mentally yell at the top of your lungs STOP. Tell yourself enough is enough and let that other more positive little inner voice take over.

So you went off your program, big deal. Just tell yourself it is a temporary thing; it's okay because it is bound to happen sooner or later. Don't allow your inner voice to beat you up. Teach it, train it, and fine tune it through positive reinforcement to become a valuable and helpful friend on your journey.

Focus

"Don't dwell on what went wrong. Instead, focus on what to do next. Spend your energies on moving forward toward finding the answer."

~Denis Whatley

The lessons taught in the majority of diet books are dreadfully misleading. Life, along with losing weight, is rarely as simple as they make it out to be. Bogus weight-loss claims and fraudulent weight-loss products target people like us who are desperate to lose weight and willing to try almost anything. Despite claims to the contrary, there are no magic bullets or effortless ways to burn fat. In fact fifty-five percent of all diet ads contain false or unsupported assertions. Unfortunately, when it comes to weight loss books, programs, and products, we can't take everything we read at face value. It's outrageous, unacceptable, frustrating and confusing. We're told about so many different methods and techniques that it makes our heads spin. It shouldn't have to be this way, but it is.

The best approach is to get back on your already proven and successful eating program. Don't waste time sorting through the vast amounts of information, hype and sometimes outrageous claims made by book authors, and companies that are just trying to get into your pockets and take your hard earned money. It's difficult because they all sound too good to be true. For the most part, the majority of the claims are just that: too good to be true.

If things are going wrong to the point where you're searching for new ideas, the best course of action is to rely on your common sense and get back to the basics. Focus on what you have known and the methods that brought you the many successes and victories you've had in the past. Don't abandon what worked for you because of a setback. The tried and true methods are always best. Getting back on track is all about focusing on your program.

You know what to do because you have already done it. If you've slipped and have to start again, then spend your energies on moving forward. That is where the answers lie.

It's impossible to Fail

"Believe and act as if it were impossible to fail."
~ *Charles Kettering*

You should never think, even for a fleeting moment, that you can't achieve your weight loss goals. It's easy to believe that's the case sometimes, especially on those occasions when you slip or cheat and feel like a complete and total failure because this is the hundredth time this has happened to you. When losing weight seems hopeless and your diet feels like an uphill battle with no relief in sight you can prevail if you want it bad enough.

If you would just pour a little gas on that spark that lies deep within you to succeed at your program, you know that spark got you going in the first place. You can ignite the spirit that created the wherewithal to start losing weight again and to get you back on track. To do this stop and consider your next move: there are consequences to any actions you may take right now. Don't allow your emotions to bring you down and make you think you're beaten by eating out of control. Try to understand where you are emotionally and take immediate counter measures. That spark that started you on your journey is still alive and deep down in your heart and soul. So find it and recapture that "I can do it" spirit once again.

You can turn this moment of possible failure into a fleeting thought that does not take root and get yourself right back on track once again. You can fan that smoldering ember that will spark your determination and turn it into a full fledged flame simply by making the next bite you place in your mouth one that is going to put you right back on your program. That magical bite will take you back to feeling good about yourself because you stopped a devastating, whirlwind spin of self destructive out of control eating that would take you far away from your weight loss goal. It all starts by *changing your attitude.* Use what you have learned over time from following your eating plan and keep doing what has worked for you. Change your thinking and start telling yourself "you can get back on track NOW!"

Once your negative inner voice has been reconditioned to this way of thinking the many bumps in the road we come upon will slowly develop into an unbeatable attitude that is set firmly in place. Making anything and everything you want from your weight loss program possible.
Back on track and all your limited thinking removed once and for all, you can become the person you want and desire to be. Armed with the right thinking and a positive attitude, you'll find any obstacles that previously held you down will be eliminated and success will take its place. You will feel a renewed sense of confidence and you will no longer doubt your abilities.

Successfully losing weight and sticking to a program is much more than just eating. It's important that you understand this. It is all about your mindset and what you think about the journey that lies ahead of you. There is so much more to it than eating certain foods and adjusting how we eat to fit an easier than done diet plan. We need to develop a new way of living and that must encompass how we think and act. In addition we must add some sort of activity levels into our plan like walking or other forms of exercise as well. Attitude alone of course isn't going to bring us to the place we want to be. But we already know what to do and we also recognize the need to incorporate some sort of exercise into our plan.

Does this mean it will be easy? Heck no or maybe the answer is yes AND no because some parts of our program will be effortless for some of us, while others will be a struggle that will cause us to doubt ourselves and our abilities.

As you are constantly being tested on all fronts, the good news is that you have the tools necessary for success in your arsenal. You just need to be constantly vigilant about any obstacle that may be placed in your way. Be ready to strike at a moment's notice to thwart off the possibility of going off your program. When you are able to do this your confidence will soar to previously unimaginable heights.

It can be tiring at times because there is so much more to losing weight than just the food we eat and how much of it we consume. There is the psychological, physical, and the nutritional aspects to losing weight.

It is important to keep this in mind and especially to remember that no matter what happens, you know you're going to get up brush yourself off and start again because you've done it before. If one weight loss method didn't work for you, you didn't give up. You mustered up the internal fortitude necessary to try another one. You bounced back and that is important to remember. You just need to reinforce that gumption and determination to keep going and build on that mental courage and soon you'll find it is impossible to fail.

Don't Get Discouraged

"Don't get discouraged, and think positive all the time. Don't get down on yourself if you lose out a couple of times. It's just a lot of hard work."

~Larisa Oleynik

The hardest part of any weight loss journey is to keep finding the motivation to continue day after day, because it can be very discouraging. Even though we have read all the diet books and have listened to all the advice to keep us on track, we still have moments when we slip, binge or go completely off our program. This can be just for one day, a few days, or for a significantly longer period of time.

When this happens, we all know it is best to get right back on our program and do it sooner rather than later. Immediately make the next bite of food we put into our mouths one that is healthy.

While this is good advice and important, there is another way of looking at these temporary slips when they do occur. Instead of beating ourselves up over losing our focus or pretending it didn't happen, we can stop and determine what made us go off-track in the first place

Analyze carefully without letting that little negative inner voice of ours judge the situation. Examine and explore only the facts and what caused you to go off-track. Really think about it until the answer comes to mind. After all, mistakes can be our best teachers.

If you're thinking this is too difficult or too demanding an exercise because you've never done this, or think that this type of self examination requires a trained professional, you couldn't be more wrong, because the reality is, we do this all the time in everyday life.

Let's say, for example, that you bake a cake and just before putting the frosting on, you taste it only to find that it tastes awful. You stop and without delay try to figure out what you did wrong that the cake came out so dreadful. You review the entire recipe and go over the process in your head, rethinking everything you did and how you did it, step by step, making sure you didn't miss anything. From start to finish you calmly scrutinize the way you made the cake to determine where or what could have possibly gone wrong.

Like the problem with the cake, instead of getting discouraged because we cheated or slipped on our eating program, all we need to do is serenely, as well as honestly, ask what was going on that made us go off track. Were you stressed, depressed, upset over something? Were you bored or angry? Were you really hungry or were your emotions controlling what happened? Your need to search for the "why" and "what" got you so disheartened that you were willing to set aside all the hard work you have done on your plan thus far.

If you take the time to examine your situation, you will gain a great deal of insight into what triggers drive you to deviate from your goals and aspirations. Next time this happens, explore what set you off, but try as hard as you can to stay positive and don't let that negative inner voice beat you up. With hard work, determination, perseverance, and learning from our mistakes we will, one day, reach our goal.

Night Time Eating*

"When it comes to eating, you can sometimes help yourself more by helping yourself less."
~Richard Armour

Are you one of those people who stick to your diet to the letter by day, only to find that as the evening progresses for some reason you turn to food? For some of us it is because of boredom, for others it could be the stress and anxiety of the day catching up with them. It's frustrating, especially, when you did so well all day only to slip once the sun goes down.

I think one thing we all must do when cravings strike is we need to determine if we are actually hungry. In other words are we experiencing actual physical hunger or are there other factors at play?

What is it that you are really feeling, that you are really craving? You should also ask yourself "what is this food really going to do for me if I eat it right now?" Sometimes the answers are tough; other times you have to confront old issues you've locked away for years that can be painful. So if the night time hours are your favorite time to raid the refrigerator after being "good" all day, you're not alone. Since rarely is this sort of eating because of an insatiable appetite for food, it is important to identify what is causing you to eat. Just stop and think about it a bit; the answers will come to you and in time you'll learn what triggers this behavior so you can avoid it.

Since we have to eat to survive, it is impossible to discontinue our relationship with food, so the next best thing is to understand its relationship with us. We need to recognize why we turn to it for comfort later in the day and examine the real reason we sought it out in the first place.

Developing a healthy relationship with food has much more to do with your attitudes toward food than it has to do with the food itself, so simply sticking to a diet or a healthy eating plan is not enough. If you can stick to your program all day then there is no reason to abandon it at night.

*NOT to be confused with "Night Eating Syndrome" an actual eating disorder.

One Success

"There is only one success – to be able to spend your life in your own way."

~Christopher Morley

Let's face it: being overweight is filled with heartache. We miss out on so many things because we simply can't, or won't, bring ourselves to participate in them. We want to; deep down we know we would enjoy ourselves, but are afraid of public opinion and ridicule. It hurts to the point of tears, yet we would never let anyone know that this is the reason that we declined their invitation. To what doesn't really matter, because we are simply not going to go and face the humiliation, the stares, the loathing looks, the ignorant ill-mannered remarks, in addition to the pointing and the laughter. It gets so old after awhile. It's tiresome, it hurts and, frankly, it seems easier to just stay behind, alone, wallowing in pity, rather than to partake of life's pleasures.

By not including ourselves in many activities, we are depriving ourselves of life experiences that could be enjoyable if we forced ourselves to go. We are also, bit by bit, chipping away at our dignity and self-esteem, fueling the fires of self-hate, negative thinking and destructive behavior patterns.

While it may take a great deal of courage to push ourselves into "doing" things and to stop from being anti-social, once we do get involved, we will find that we enjoy being out and about, totally caught up in the moment and the event. It's all about you and how you spend your life.

Once You Label Me

"Once you label me, you negate me."

~Soren Kierkegaard

Once you decide a certain food is "bad" for you, like ice cream, for example, something very predictable begins formulating in your mind. As absurd as it is, labeling something bad has a way of making us think about it more. Suddenly, this awful food appears in front of us everywhere we go and it happens to be everywhere we look. It becomes unavoidable and starts taking root in our minds so even our thoughts are drawn to it.

The very thing we were attempting to avoid by telling ourselves that a certain food is bad for us is what we are now thinking about subconsciously repeatedly. From time to time it even seems to call our name. When it does that, it's hopeless because we will start to crave it more than when we weren't trying to avoid it. Suddenly we are out of control until we satisfy our desire for it.

Our normal self control and the ability to make healthy choices are substituted with the contemplation of bingeing. Once manifested, we can no longer hear our sensible side that keeps us on track to our weight loss goals. The capacity to choose, our self-awareness of what we're doing and the quantity of food we should be eating diminishes with every passing moment.

We become so distracted that the negative impact of all this won't hit us until later when we come back to our senses. Consider making all foods neutral. Don't divide foods into "good" and "bad." It is not going to help you on your weight-loss journey.

Mr. Temptation

"Opportunity may knock only once, but temptation leans on the doorbell."

~Author unknown

It surely seems that temptation leans on that ole doorbell a lot, doesn't it? It constantly tries to lead us off-course from losing weight and reaching our ideal goal, placing difficult hurdles along the way at every opportunity.

One of the biggest temptations we face daily is the choice of food to eat on our program. You're not going to lose weight eating double pound hamburgers, with enhanced size fries and a jumbo soft drink. Commercials for the wrong food choices are everywhere we look: TV, magazines, newspaper ads, we even hear them on the radio. They constantly bombard us, all the while trying to persuade us that their product is the best, most satisfying, filling and enjoyable. Everyone always look so happy in those ads. Candy, fast food, TV dinners, meals out of a box, all these and more are relentlessly beckoning us to buy them, all the while saying it's okay to take the decision process away from us.

In addition to food ads, there are the many social gatherings we encounter which are far worse than any commercial. Co-workers, friends or family members want to meet you somewhere to eat. All make an effort to convince you that it's okay to have this or that food just this one time. Although these people may have good intentions and care for you, statements like "don't worry about your diet just this once," aren't the type of encouragement you need to hear.

The reality is, temptation leans on the doorbell much more often than we would like when faced with a choice; we have an obligation to ourselves to continually make an effort to select what is going to keep us heading towards achieving the goals we desire. "Healthy alternatives" need to be in the forefront of our mind all the time to help us at any turn where temptation might lurk.

Learn to Relax

"Your mind will answer most questions if you learn to relax and wait for the answer"

~William S. Burroughs

When you are on a weight loss program, if you encounter stress and don't take measures to release it, you could trigger an emotional eating frenzy that will only lead to weight gain. It will raise your stress levels even more, as well as diminish your capacity to be level-headed and stay in control of your eating as you attempt to stay on track with your program.

The explanation as to why we eat out of emotions like stress is because usually our reaction to stress is to sit and stew in our frustration and anger. This sends a hormonal signal to replenish our nutritional stores. So there is actually a clinical reason we eat out of frustration. It's not totally our fault.

If that isn't bad enough, the "fuel" our muscles need during this fight is sugar and it's the prime reason that when our stress levels are increased we crave carbohydrates. High levels of sugar and insulin set the stage for the body to store fat. You can see from this that stress can open a real can of worms for us. As a result, eating becomes the activity that relieves the stress. It's easy to do and it's comforting."

As much as we would like to blame all our weight gain on stress and eating out of emotion, repeating this response over time can actually become a habit, one that's encouraged by brain chemistry.

So we need to make a change to overcome this cycle of events. We need to take time out when stressed, instead of eating out of emotion. We have to teach ourselves to take a deep breath, count to ten, then just relax and let all our anxiety pass. Devoting time to relaxation in fact works much like exercise to produce brain chemicals that counter the effects of stress. The answers are there if you want them: just relax.

Incredible Things

"When you wholeheartedly adopt a "with all your heart" attitude and go all out with the positive principle, you can do incredible things"

~Norman Vincent Peale

There is a big difference between starting a weight loss journey and starting a diet. A weight loss journey is a lifetime approach to better over-all health. It is a way of life that we must create and accept for ourselves. It is the establishment of new, permanent changes in our minds by establishing new habits, behaviors and thinking.

A diet is a temporary fix filled with feelings of being deprived and being disappointed, in addition to it being a constant struggle with ourselves.

Once you decide to commence on a weight loss journey that will be for the rest of your life. There will be a new flame burning deep within your soul crying out "there is no stopping me now!" Your normally negative inner voice will be substituted with one that will shout approval with immense conviction. You will feel stronger emotionally, radiating a cloud of confidence and a sense of well being.

A reason must exist for you to succeed; you need to find a motivation to drive you, one that burns within your heart. If you do, you'll be amazed at the difference in the way you'll feel about your journey this time around compared to any previous attempts.

I Can't Take It Anymore!

"I'm sick and tired of being sick and tired."

~Fannie Lou Hamer

"I'm sick and tired of dieting and trying to lose weight. I'm sick of it! I simply can't take it anymore!"

I am sure you have cried this phrase with real tears streaming down your face, pleading with a higher power to help you. Poor us! Oh the troubles, trials, tribulations and the struggles we face everyday. What a pity, what a shame…. You're sick of it already and who blames you?

Well, for one thing, it's evident that you do. Heck, we've all done it. Sometimes it's helpful to have a good old-fashioned cry and get out our frustrations. Except next time we need to gain control over this situation when it happens. We can make it to where we don't have to go down this path again and again. Today we can make things better starting right now. We have 86,400 seconds to use constructively ahead of us each day. We have the time and we know what must be done to lose the weight. Clearly it's not all about knowledge, because we know what we have to do to lose weight. What we really need to do is to put that know-how into action and do it.

If your are sick of trying to lose weight, then get determined to succeed and end this emotional roller coaster ride once and for all. Stop hoping that you might lose weight or that maybe you'll succeed today, and make it happen. The deck is not as stacked against you as you may think. If you eat right and are determined not to give in when your program is not going the way you'd like it to, you will lose weight, and you will reach your goal. If you continue to eat right, you will remain at your goal weight for the rest of your life. This can happen even if you have a huge amount of weight to lose and a long road ahead of you to get there.

By learning to cope with our challenges, rather than running from them to food that will only add to your unhappiness, you will have taken a major step towards being victorious, this day, and all future days.

For us, unfortunately, the struggle really never ends. Unlike a smoker or alcoholic who doesn't need their addiction to survive, we must continue to use food to fuel our bodies. We cannot avoid eating and, as a result, must always continue a healthy weight loss eating program or lose control. But victory can be ours if we just stop being "sick and tired of being tired" of it all and get used to the fact that we must continue our fight for life. We will succeed only if we stop blaming ourselves and focus on making things better one second at a time.

Feeling Sad

"The greatness comes not when things go always good for you. But the greatness comes when you're really tested, when you take some knocks, some disappointments, when sadness comes. Because only if you've been in the deepest valley can you ever know how magnificent it is to be on the highest mountain."

~Richard Nixon

At times it may feel as though you're the only person in the world who is having difficulty losing weight. Just about everyone you know seems to have their program together, along with their exercise, eating healthy, cutting calories and losing weight while you are dying inside. It may look as if the battle of the bulge is winning in your life, but you have the power to overcome these feelings.

The reality is that there isn't a single person who hasn't experienced these feelings while dieting. This leads to a sense of loneliness and isolation, usually because we have fewer confidants in our lives and feel disconnected from most people we know. There is nothing more torturous than needing support or just someone who will listen or to whom we can vent.

When discontentment is set into motion because of our lack of progress on our program, and the unhappiness we experience towards ourselves begins, we believe we are a failure by not meeting our own preset expectations. It is no exaggeration to say many of us put ourselves through a nightmare of misery judging ourselves like this. Once self-doubt and low esteem manifest themselves, food softly calls our name, making empty promises that it is all right to have a binge fest or to treat ourselves to anything we desire; furthermore, if we do, we'll feel better and our anxieties will disappear.

We know from experience that this is not the case. We've traveled that path too many times to fall for that destructive inner voice of ours, whose only intention is to distract us from our weight loss goals. It may feel that you're the only person in the world who is having difficulty losing weight. However you are not alone.

One Giant Step That Does It

"There is no one giant step that does it. It's a lot of little steps."

~Peter A. Cohen

Anyone who has any amount of weight to lose knows that there is no magic pill, shot, diet drink or bar that you can take and then sit back and have the pounds melt away, especially while you sleep, like many products claim.

The fact is, it's hard to lose weight. It takes effort and discipline. It's a daily struggle, but over time, your actions become new life-style habits and eventually you can and will reach your goal.

But because we live in an "I want it now" society, it makes losing weight more problematic for us. We are so used to having it "right now" with drive-in windows, instant film processing, and movies on demand, fast food restaurants, and microwave dinners. We are susceptible to buying into those instant weight loss ads and programs. We want something that will just "do it" for us because we are tired of the daily battle that we must fight to lose even a pound or two a week. We dream of the day that something will come along that will actually work and all our excess fat will be gone.

Maybe someday there will be something that can be done to help make it easier or more effortless to lose weight, but until then we need to continue to take the steps that will get us to our ultimate goal. Its hard work, but what things in life aren't?

These steps don't have to be drastic, giant leaps. They can be an accumulation of many little things. It is the little steps that will keep adding up. Walk up the stairs instead of taking the elevator, or try not to get the closest parking space to the door next time you go shopping. Try parking farther out and do a little extra walking. How about leaving food on your plate instead of finishing it? Little steps… first one, then two, then as you become comfortable with them, add another and another until you have added a lot of little steps that take you right to your dreams.

Failure is an Opportunity

"Failure is the opportunity to begin again more intelligently."

~ Henry Ford

We all know what it is like to struggle with our weight. Some of us have been doing it all our lives. It is a fight we often think we can't win, to the point of disappointment, frustration and despair. We feel defeated because, in time, there seems to come a point, while on our journey of losing weight and eating healthier, that we stumble and go off our eating program. Some call it cheating, others will tell you that they slipped, pigged out, or binged. Whatever people label the situation; it is devastating and sends us on a whirlwind of self-destruction.

It is at this instant that we feel like a failure and as a result often become disheartened and lose sight of our goal and, more important, we lose sight of what we have accomplished thus far. We begin to feel sorry for ourselves and wish that the battle over losing weight didn't take so much exertion, effort and energy to achieve. Our confidence deteriorates quickly and our belief that we can accomplish our goals diminishes to the point that we start to feel sorry for ourselves and ask rhetorically "why me". Why is this so difficult? Why can't I lose more? Why does this take so long? Why, why, why.

There is no doubt that a setback, whether it be minor, temporary, a plateau or a major binge fest, hurts. It cuts deep into our motivation and desire to continue the battle another day. But setbacks are not failures unless we allow them to be. They aren't failures unless we convince ourselves they are.

Look at them realistically: they are an opportunity of renewed faith, a new beginning, if you will. They are a chance to start over again, instead of an excuse to wallow in self pity and go further off our goals.

You need to find the strength inside of you when these setbacks occur, and they will. Use positive self talk and reinforcement instead of negative or "stinking thinking." You will succeed quickly towards getting back on track if you do. You should be as kind to yourself as you would a dear friend who needs your advice and council. You have to be supportive and remind yourself how far you've come on your journey instead of beating yourself up. You grasp the fact that one setback is not going to define your past achievements or future goals. Use this as an opportunity to retrain your thinking.

Enlightenment

"The moment of enlightenment is when a person's dreams of possibilities become images of probabilities."

~Vic Braden

When the time comes that you decide to get back on track and get going again on losing weight, it is also that instance when you should take action on your dream and turn it into a probability. You know what I mean: when that light bulb goes off in your head and your dream of losing weight is born again. This flash of enlightenment is when you need to act and make it all happen. It is when your attitude and belief is at its utmost, as is your enthusiasm, desire and determination.

When you take your first step on what can be a long, arduous journey, be deliberate in your expectations of what you want to achieve. It is unrealistic expectations and lack of preparation that are the most common causes of failure, so now that you have a dream, turn it into a reality, but don't set yourself up for failure by selecting goals that you can't reach.

Prepare yourself and be truthful with yourself, asking "why now?" Think what is it that made you decide to get going again and do you really want to do it. Start thinking thin twenty-four hours a day, visualizing yourself at the weight you want to be. Since results are our guru, take notice along your journey to observe any changes and use them to keep you going.

Old Worn Out Excuses

"Excuses are the nails used to build a house of failure."

~ Don Wilder and Bill Rechin

Excuses, excuses, excuses. We all have them. We all use some of them so much that they have long been worn-out and the people you know are tired of hearing them over and over again. Excuses like:

"Right after the holidays I will join a gym."
"I am going to buy a treadmill the next time I see one on sale."
"Once it cools off, I'll start walking."
"Once it starts warming up, I'll start swimming."
"I am going to make sure I drink eight glasses of water every day."
"It's not fair! I don't eat THAT much!"
"I am so tired of having to be on a diet!!!!!!!"
"Diets just don't work."
"It's so hard . . . to lose weight."
"I'm happy with myself just the way I am."

It's time to stop justifying reasons that are designed to prevent you from achieving what you desire from your program and what you want out of life. It is time to put these excuses behind you and take responsibility for making healthy choices again. You need to stop playing these worn-out excuses over and over in your mind and do what is required to stick to your eating plan once and for all. Doing this requires patience and persistence.
It requires us to get back up when we fall down.
It requires us to make our goal a priority.
It requires not having a half-hearted attitude.

But most of all, it requires us to really WANT to do it.

The Longer You Wait

"The longer you wait to decide what you want to do, the more time you're wasting. It's up to you to want something so badly that your passion shows through in your actions. Your actions, not your words, will do the shouting for you."

~ Derek Jeter

Are you like many people who are sick and tired of constantly watching their weight or being on a diet? Or are you on an eating plan and doing well for a while, then for no good reason, fall off the wagon, get so discouraged, and so disappointed that you just throw in the towel and quit?

That is when the frustration and anger with yourself begins. That is when you need to direct your attention to you, instead of allowing your program to be set on the back burner. You need to make up your mind to get back on track again, and right away at that, because the longer you wait to decide what you want to do about your eating plan, and getting back on track, the more disappointment and heartache you will experience. If you do not decide right away you will begin a downward spiral that will take even more effort to pull yourself out. You need to start feeling that spark in your heart again called hope. Once it ignites, it is hard to put out and will carry you a long way towards your goals. It will be the catalyst that will get you moving again, revitalizing your effort and determination once more, making you feel re-energized about your weight loss and long-term healthier lifestyle changes.

There is hardly a single person who has not been down this road, so believe me, you are not alone. It is up to you to regain that spark and that commitment you made to yourself so that you can once again move forward.

Don't put a lot of emphasis right now on regarding a number you see on the scale. If you set aside your program for a while, the number on the scale will go up, and seeing it could cause you to start the cycle of wanting to give up again. Focus, instead, on taking care of you by eating right. Make the correct choices that will get you closer to where you want to be again and stay active – both mentally and physically. It will be inspiring and will motivate you again as you experience more and more progress! It will encourage you to believe in yourself and your goals again. Once you believe in yourself and clear your mind of any defeatist attitudes, anything I possible . . . including losing weight.

Doubt Whom You Will

"Doubt whom you will, but never yourself."

~ *Christine Bovee*

When you're dieting, occasionally it is difficult to find the energy, discipline and desire to stay on your eating program everyday. At times it just seems like a never-ending battle. In fact, most people who are overweight have a life history of being overweight and are tired of constantly struggling to stay in control.

This can be very disheartening to the point that you feel, "I'm never going to do this!" All the work and effort seems futile. Any doubts concerning our chances of succeeding can bring about other feelings like disappointment, self-disgust and shame. Doubt, simply put, inwardly causes something to leave us. It creates that ever-so-familiar sinking feeling in the pit of our stomach, which turns our despair into anger, which is of course always pointed at us.

It is this self-doubt that we need to remove from our thought process. After all, we know we can lose weight even if we have to repeat the process over and over to finally get it to sink in. Positive thoughts generate positive results.

Choice

"It's so hard when I have to, and so easy when I want to."

~Sondra Anice Barnes

Funny, how when we 'want' to do something it is accomplished so easily. When losing weight, if it is your own convictions that compel you, then you will find that the road to success is comprised of less bumps along the way, less obstacles to overcome and less choices in which direction to travel.

On the other hand, if your motivation to lose weight is because your doctor told you to do it, or your partner, spouse, significant other, or some other reason except for your own internalized sureness, you're not going to find the journey down any road a pleasant one.

Your journey will be chock-full of side roads and paths trying to divert and redirect you from the main road. There will be more obstacles and hurdles to defeat you, but you must have the determination and willpower to overcome them. It will be difficult, exhausting and emotionally draining.

When the time is right to lose weight, it must be your choice. It can't be because of someone else's influence; it must be entirely your idea. Your purpose must be clear to you, your goals set and realistic, your expectations clear, and your focus intense.

This is your journey to travel and yours alone. It will be long, tedious and disheartening at times, so you need to be prepared and anticipate what you will encounter along the way. Easy? Not by a long shot, but as long as it is your choice, then success awaits you at the end of that road.

Capable Hands

"You need to accept the fact that from this moment on, you're in Capable hands – yours."

~Zig Ziglar

Ever sit alone feeling sorry for yourself, wanting a little sympathy? Perhaps you've sat crying, cursing the world asking "Why Me"? Why can't I lose weight? Why am I fat? Why is life so hard? Why, why, why? Or maybe you wish that you could somehow magically lose weight, or pray to a divine force to give you some sort of super-human willpower so that you can stay on track and achieve your goals, putting your future and weight loss success in a higher power's capable hands. Maybe you've dreamt that you could just go into a long fairy tale-like sleep, wake up and you're thin. Or take some magic weight loss pill.

Wishing and dreaming is okay for some things but losing weight is not one of them. Feeling sorry for your self isn't healthy either, and your aspiration to lose weight is all about health, so the two go hand in hand. We put the weight on, so it is up to us to take it off.

We need to recognize the fact, that, throughout the years we have obtained a wealth of knowledge when it comes to losing weight and know what we need to do to lose it. Let's face it; people with a large amount of weight to lose have probably read every book on weight loss or close to it. We know more about diets, dieting, weight loss programs, calorie counting, fat contents, carbohydrates and what really works or doesn't work than most doctors. We understand the mechanics and know the techniques to succeed.

You may have failed many times and it's hard trying over and over again to lose weight. But you have to do it again, only this time you need to accept the fact that from this moment on, you're in capable hands – yours. Once you believe this in your heart you're on your way to succeeding and keeping the weight off.

Can't

"If someone says can't, that shows you what to do."

~John Cage

When you're struggling to lose weight, the word "can't" often emerges in your mind, or there is someone who tries to burst your bubble by telling you all kinds of stories about people they know who tried this or that and failed at it. It's almost like they don't want you to succeed.

Whether you think you can't or are told you can't, if you take ownership of that thought, you will be derailed off your weight loss program. Any feelings of self-worth and self-esteem you have left will become compromised, as well as losing your determination, devotion and passion to fight another day. That is how influential and powerful the word "can't" is. Like a magic elixir, the word "can't" is so persuasive, it redefines your ability to focus on what is important to you. It reshapes your entire thought process and is so compelling that it will change your capacity to achieve success in anything you try or desire.

Once you develop a plan of action to lose weight, or have an aspiration of something you want to do or start on, stick with it. Don't permit anyone to advise you except for someone who is successful at whatever it is you want to do, or has accomplished what you're planning to undertake. People who tell you that you can't do something are more often than not completely incorrect.

These cynics rarely, if ever, have carried out anything of significance in their own lives, and yet they have the nerve to tell you what you can or cannot achieve with yours. Imagine if people like Edison listened to the many individuals who told him he was wasting his time trying to invent the light bulb. Or the Wright brothers, if they listened to all the doubting Thomas's when they were told over and over again that they would never fly.

If you have an idea, a plan of action and someone insists that it can't be done, use their discouraging reasoning as your personal roadmap of exactly what you should be doing and on what you should be focusing. As long as your goals and dreams are realistic, in that they are reachable, you must have faith in your ability to achieve them. Your weight loss success or accomplishing any goal or something you want to do, all start deep within you. It all begins with the single notion that you can and will accept the challenge before you, and become the instrument to initiate the changes that need to be made to do it. There is no such word as can't *"just keep doing it and it will get done!"*

A New Day

**"No one can go back and make a brand new start. Anyone can start from now and
make a brand new ending."**

~Unknown

We can't go back in time and start over again if we have slipped, cheated, gained weight, or gone off our eating program, but that doesn't mean that we have to give up because of it either. We all have moments when we want to just throw in the towel, but at least we are always given the opportunity to start over from right now and re-write how our day will end.

We can choose to continue to be out of control and allow ourselves to binge, until we're so stuffed we feel sick. All the while, we beat ourselves to a pulp mentally, internalizing what a failure we are. Or we can immediately stop this destructive process and get back on our diet or healthy eating program.

Losing weight is hard work! As I have said before, it requires patience and, most of all, persistence. It necessitates that you get back up when you fall and make your weight loss goals your main priority at that moment in time. You need to get right back on your program by making the next bite you put in your mouth one that is a healthy choice and one that is on your plan. I call it, "taking a bite at a time."™

Patience is hard when it comes to losing weight, because being on a diet can be such a long journey to undertake. It gets discouraging at times to the point that you don't feel like fighting another day to stay on your plan. A lot of this has to do with us living in an "I want it now" society mind-set. Drive-through restaurants, one-hour photo processing, instant printing, express mail service, oil changes while you wait, the list is endless.

The habits we have developed from years of abusing our bodies are not going to go away quickly. We must be conscious of them and overcome them through a keener sense of what we are doing when it comes to food. It takes time to actually see this, however, by keeping a food journal of everything we eat. This consciousness will eventually become a new way of eating and forming good habits.
Expecting too much too fast will only bring disappointment. We aren't going to become a completely different person overnight. Our new day is an opportunity to persist and do well, eventually getting our destination.

As I See It

"As I see it, every day you do one of two things: Build health or produce disease in yourself."

~Adelle Davis

Every day in life is a clean slate in which we are given an opportunity to start afresh. It is truly a unique gift. If we use it wisely, we can do some amazing things with it.

When it comes to losing weight and promoting our health, we can use this opportunity to not only get us closer to our dieting goals, but to encourage a more complete and healthier us. We can focus on the important issues that affect people who need to lose weight, mainly our health.

According to a study published September 26, 2006, in the medical journal *Critical Care*, having diabetes, for instance, increases one's chances of developing a critical illness and/or dying early; obesity alone does not. And obese people suffer more from diabetes than any other group of people.

So it is important that we don't only concentrate on losing weight and nothing else; we must also find the courage to face any medical issues we need to deal with as well.

Many people who have large amounts of weight to lose avoid doctors. This is because early childhood memories of doctor visits were met by physicians that did not really understand the issues we faced and were not compassionate to our needs or feelings.

But we're getting older now, and it's time to put those childhood fears behind us and confront whatever medical conditions we may have head on.

It is essential to develop healthier habits, which encompasses not only losing weight, but taking care of yourself, and that is not a one-time activity. It needs to be the focal point of your daily existence so that you can live a fruitful tomorrow. Of course you can choose not to be responsible for yourself medically, only concentrating on your weight, but the two go hand in hand.

There is so much work to be done to take back our lives and all the years of abuse and neglect that we have inflicted on ourselves. It takes such an enormous effort, that some days we don't know if we can continue on, but we must. Frankly, it's a struggle that, for many, the odds are against you.

If we combine our weight loss efforts, however, along with taking care of ourselves by adopting a new way of thinking and simply staying on top of them both for the rest of our lives, then we will have the quality of life that we can enjoy well into the future.

A Single Defeat

"Never confuse a single defeat with a final defeat"

~ F. Scott Fitzgerald

For some unknown reason, we can be doing fantastic on our diet or healthy eating program, then without a second's notice we lose complete control and go on a binge. Something or someone triggers a deep emotional response. We dive into a panicked state of mind where we start to make irrational decisions regarding our food intake and consumption.

You know how to gain weight; that part is easy, but by now you are also experts at losing weight as well. You have all the knowledge you require from years of experience on how to shed those extra pounds. It is during these times that we need to kick in all that know-how and experience to get us back on track. Normally when we have a setback like this, what is lacking is our way of thinking about our weight loss program. It is our emotional state that determines our successes, our temporary defeats and failures.

We all know that there is so much more to weight loss than just eating, so it is essential to be deliberate on how we communicate with ourselves. Our thoughts, feelings, ideas, beliefs, values, moods, and the way we see ourselves, plus our expectations, will seriously manipulate our outcomes if we continue to think negatively. Simply stated, if you tell yourself you are big, fat, and disgusting, you'll most likely keep on overeating because you're creating a self-fulfilling prophecy.

If you continue to do what you've always done, you'll get what you've always got. Small changes in your habits and beliefs will result in the permanent changes you would like for better health and weight loss. Always be aware of your emotional state when you eat. If you are stressed from the day or have unconstructive negative feelings floating around in your head, or you feel angry, bored, depressed, or frustrated, then take a time out. Uses self-talk to place your self in a calmer mood, before feeding these emotions. Redirect your focus away from food and do something else before you actually begin your meal until you are more composed.

If you slip up along the way and this causes you to feel defeated, that is not an excuse to spiral out of control and lose all hope. As long as you continue the battle you will achieve the results you want.

People Who Live in a Dream World

"There are some people, who live in a dream world, and there are some who face reality; and then there are those who turn one into the other."

~Beecher Douglas Everett

Enough of the snake oil already! Any diet, diet supplement, weight loss book or eating program that promises dramatic results is nothing but a sham. If you believe their hype, then you're living in a dream world, because while some may produce results, none will last long.

It is because we are so worn out from the constant struggle to lose weight, that these quick fix shams even appeal to us. We are tired of battling the ever-so-familiar and overwhelming feelings of having to stay on track and stick to a healthier eating plan, which we must, even when we want to eat uncontrollably.

These nonsense products exist because they appeal to our most intimate inner thoughts and fears, in addition to our worries about failing. They promise fast, immediate and easy results so we don't have to continue down that long wearisome road that we must travel to achieve our weight loss goals. It is how we get hooked and tempted to abandon everything that we have learned about sensible and healthy eating.

We need to stop impatiently pursuing losing weight. Despite what quick-weight-loss books or products may say, the only sensible way to lose weight and maintain a healthy weight permanently is to eat less and balance your food intake with physical activity. It is a long journey, so we have to adopt the fact that it is going to take time to reach our goal.

In addition, we need to find the wherewithal to go the distance, and face the reality of this being a lifetime healthy eating program. Sure we can dream of much less demanding lifestyle changes, such as exercise and diet. We can fantasize about quick fixes and magical pills that make you lose weight without dieting while you sleep, and other such nonsense, but it is essential to take these dreams and work at turning them into tangible realities.

It's tough when things aren't going as quickly as we think they should. It's all about being patient and maintaining self-control when these feelings begin, that we're not losing weight rapidly enough. It's all about taking charge of our attitude and building our self-esteem while using our common sense.

There are more than fifty individual dietary supplements and more than one hundred twenty-five commercial combination products that are available for weight loss. Combine that with hundreds of weight loss and diet books, infomercials, cabbage soup and other such magic bullet soup diets, and it is easy to see how we could be drawn in by their numerous false hopes and promises.

You really have to want to lose weight and forget the oxymoron of any diet being quick and easy. You should face the concept that you will never, ever again in your life be able to eat anything you want and there is no effortless anything on this planet that is going to make you lose weight without you working for it. That's a hard reality and a lot of people aren't going to make it because of that, but if you really, really want to lose weight, you can do it.

Choices, Choices, Choices

"The future is not a result of choices among alternative paths offered by the present, but a place that is created—created first in the mind and will, created next in activity. The future is not some place we are going to, but one we are creating. The paths are not to be found, but made, and the activity of making them, changes both the maker and the destination."

~Anonymous quote

Losing weight is a long journey made up of constant choices. The great thing about these choices is that you have the power and the ability to determine their outcome. Whatever your choice is when you make it, you're the one who has to live with its end result. Positive or negative, there is still a consequence to be paid based on your decision. If temptation strikes, take a deep breath and think for a moment about the outcome of your choice before you finalize your decision.

Today, choose to take care of yourself along with creating your future doing it. Spend some time alone and think of what a wonderful person you are. You are unique, and one of a kind. Take care of yourself; there will never be another you.

Attitude

"I have reached a point in my life where I understand the pain and the challenges; and my attitude is one of standing up with open arms to meet them all."

~Myrlie Evers

Losing weight for countless numbers of people is easy, but it is a familiar, as well as a predictable, statistic that keeping the weight off is difficult, at best, for everyone.

Fighting to keep off the pounds gets discouraging, but you can beat the odds with a very powerful weapon even fewer people are able to draw on, and that is your attitude. The right attitude will keep you on track and moving toward your goal. It will get you back on your path if you slip up, falter, or have difficulties, and it will sustain you when all your hope, determination and will to carry on seem lost.

Staying motivated is a huge dilemma, because reaching our goal weight and keeping those lost pounds off is such an arduous task. The road to our goal is so long that sometimes we lose sight of the finish line. This is especially true if we're struggling just to maintain the weight we've lost.

Attitude is everything, though; if you can change your thoughts, you can change the degree of progress and success that you will achieve. By changing the way you think, you will advance much quicker than you are capable of ever achieving by physical action and diet alone.

The trick is to understand the struggle, challenges and pain you have. Deal with it, in addition to removing the emotion out of your eating plan to keep you on track. But whatever you do, keep in mind the initial passion that motivated you to embark on your weight loss journey. It is that zeal, eagerness and enthusiasm that you need to embrace yet again to keep you going.

Simply stated, change your point of view; open your arms to meet whatever difficulties or obstacles are thrown your way. Have a positive attitude and it will be easier to continue your commitment to eat and live a healthier lifestyle. Doing this will result in weight loss – you can make a difference if you're struggling. It's all in your attitude.

The Fear of Failure

"Don't fear failure so much that you refuse to try new things. The saddest summary of a life contains three descriptions: could have, might have, and should have."

~Louis E. Boone

People who are on a diet or healthy eating program have setbacks. They are an inevitable fact of life for us, but too often we look upon these setbacks as failures.

A setback is not an easy road from which to pick yourself up and continue to travel. It is extremely exasperating and frustrating. We need to be patient; a healthy weight loss plan is not a diet or a race. It is a complete lifestyle change, more like a journey with many roads, paths, and hurdles to overcome. There will be countless obstacles in our way, steps to go up, hills to climb and mountains to scale. So we prepare for them, because this journey is one that we will be traveling for a long time. As such, speed is not important; the only thing that matters is reaching our destination – goal weight.

If we have a few slip-ups here and there along the way, that doesn't mean that we have failed. We shouldn't fear getting off-track every now and then, because as long as you get back on your program, nothing is preventing you from reaching your goal.

When we lose our direction and focus for a short time, we need to re-establish where we want to go and make the next bite we take a healthy choice that will take us there.

Stop any negative messages in your head before they take root, control your emotions and replace them with positive ones.

The reality is your mindset is the only thing that stands between you, and the things that you want to achieve in life. If you want to continue losing weight, and want it bad enough, you will do the work that is required to get back on track.

The worst thing we could ever do is to be so fearful of failure that we don't keep trying. Because as long as we keep getting up, dusting ourselves off and continuing on, we will have no failures.

Don't ever give up because all you'll end up with is a bunch of could have, might have and should haves left in your life, along with a lot of wasted time that may well have been spent doing what had to be done.

Just keep on getting up when you fall. Don't be discouraged. If it doesn't happen this week, it will occur next week if you just keep working at it. Nobody's perfect, and the only difference between success and failure is getting up one more time, every time. Extend the same understanding of having a bad day or a bump in the road to yourself, as you would do for others, and stop holding yourself to a different set of weight loss standards. We're all in this together.

We Grow Because We Struggle

"We grow because we struggle, we learn and overcome."

~RobertAllen

Losing weight is tough enough without us making it more complicated. We don't deliberately set out to make our path difficult, but somehow, somewhere along our journey, we got the notion in our head that if we struggle, we will succeed in our quest and achieve our goals. It's kind of like the old saying when it comes to exercise "it has to hurt to be beneficial". People say this all the time, but it simply is not true. Neither does the amount of struggle we experience when dieting or eating healthier, equate to the amount of our future successes. Just because losing weight is demanding, it doesn't mean we have to choose the hardest road possible to achieve it.

The hard road is when we encounter a setback which happens from time to time, or we don't lose weight fast enough and we switch on this mode of self-defeating behavior. We focus on our faults and shortcomings instead of yesterday's victories.

If you slipped, cheated, or had a weight gain, that doesn't mean that you have to exchange blows with yourself. We often become our own worst enemy with this self-defeating attitude. Over time, and not much of it, it becomes a kind of self-sabotage where we begin to focus on our shortcomings and lack of progress, and then end up feeling worse and worse. Soon we start to feel sorry for ourselves and before we know it, we're feeding our out-of-control emotions.

Learning is the key to ending this vicious cycle. If we focus on everything we know about a diet or eating plan and healthy choices, we will continue to realize positive results. If you feel you'll never win, that is because struggling to lose weight is a misplaced battle.

Do it differently this time around to win "the struggle." Relax. Take it slow. After all, it took time to put that weight on and it is going to take time to take it off. Take small steps towards that finish line and learn to be patient with yourself. We must give up the fighting with that 'person' in our head who hates us, and put a stop to our negative self-destructive thinking. We must stop asking "why me" and continue forging forward toward our goals.

Look, we know everything there is about dieting, probably more than most doctors because we have been doing it so long. We are knowledgeable about counting calories and avoiding trans- fats. We exercise, keep food logs, count carbohydrates and cholesterol. We know what we should eat and how much of it in order to lose weight. We are the authorities on healthy choices; we are nutrition experts, just without the formal training and degrees. We can overcome this and put an end to our weight loss struggle by simply, 'doing' whatever it takes to do it.

Why Me?

"But there is suffering in life, and there are defeats. No one can avoid them. But it's better to lose some of the battles in the struggles for your dreams than to be defeated without ever knowing what you're fighting for."

~Paulo Coelho

Why me? – a very common question asked by people who struggle with their weight and are tormented by it. Why have I been singled out to endure this suffering and have to struggle so much?

The questions we ask ourselves, "Why me? Why am I this way?" Or "What have I done to deserve being this? What is the purpose of me having to suffer so much?" are extremely intense questions we often ask with tears streaming down our faces.

Our weight is so visible and reality-based that life can be extremely tough on us. Mean spirited people can destroy our egos with one glaring look of disgust or a snide remark. A child pointing and laughing at us can be all it takes to bring us to tears, but the question "why me?" nonetheless remains unanswered and may ultimately be unanswerable.

Unfortunately, good people like us, do not always win. Life isn't fair and certainly is not a bowl of cherries. Add being obese to the mix and it's an utter living hell. The torment, the pain, the struggle we must put up with would devastate the toughest of normal sized people.

It's safe to say "the one thing we should learn from experience is that we do not learn from experience." History speaks for itself and we all have cried those "why me?" tears too many times. It does not, however, seem to have changed much deep down inside us. With predictable consistency, we continue allowing this negative behavior to manifest itself throughout our weight loss journey. Doing this injures our ego, brings on bouts of depression, along with a defeatist attitude toward our weight loss dreams and goals.

Being human means that we can't avoid these stumbling blocks, that we are going to fail from time to time and that we are going to cry "why me?" It's best to come to this understanding now, accepting it as fact, so when the day comes you'll know what you're fighting for.

You Too Can Be Great

"Keep away from people who try to belittle your ambitions. Small people always do that, but the really great make you feel that you, too, can become great."

~ Mark Twain

Just because you have tried losing weight before and didn't reach your goal, that doesn't mean through persistence you won't accomplish it. How many times have you started over? How many times have you told friends and family this time you're going to do it?

Then out of the blue you join a health spa or a weight loss support group like T.O.P.S., Overeaters Anonymous, Weight Watchers, or start a healthy eating program and you let everyone know, thinking they will encourage you and support your efforts. Maybe they will even remind you to stay true to your program and help keep you on track if you start to deviate from your plan.

Instead you're met with indifference and a total lack of enthusiasm because your friends and family have heard it all from you countless times before. In fact, so many times that their belief level and faith in you to "do it" this time around isn't there.

Sometimes it is best to not tell people your plans, especially if they won't be supportive and encouraging of your plan to lose weight. Finding a support system is critical to long-term weight loss. Whether you join a group such as T.O.P.S., Overeaters Anonymous, Weight Watchers, or do something else, it's beneficial to share your highs and lows with people who can relate with your struggle. These same people can also be a valuable source of new ideas and strategies. Like-minded people who share your enthusiasm and have similar goals and dreams understand what it takes to lose weight. By turning to them, you know you're not alone and together, you too, can become great.

You Can Succeed

"You can succeed if nobody else believes it, but you will never succeed if you don't believe it yourself."

~William De Montaigne

Beware of the doubting Thomas in your head who says you won't succeed in your attempt to lose weight because you've tried it a hundred times before.

As long as you can see yourself accomplishing your weight loss goal and your objective is realistic, there is no stopping you. If you can't see yourself at your goal weight – then do it today by not only seeing it, but believing it as well.

To lose weight, it certainly isn't something that you have to 'believe in' for it to achieve results. However, if you don't, your journey will be short lived and filled with disappointment.

It is more likely than not that you will end up going back to your old eating and exercise habits, since your thoughts do not match your actions by not presuming you can succeed. When you change your thoughts to insist on success, you will be so much closer to your goal than you could ever get by actions alone.

So if you have any doubt or don't believe you can do it, then the first thing you need to do is silence the critic within you because you'll never succeed if you don't believe it yourself.

You Can Have Big Plans

"You can have big plans, but it's the small choices that have the greatest power. They draw us toward the future we want to create."

~ Robert Cooper

When you take that first step toward losing weight, you've decided that enough is enough. You have reached that point in time when you're tired of gaining weight and all you want is to be like everyone else. All you want is to go unnoticed in a room because you fit in and for once aren't the biggest person there.

When this day comes, it is okay to dream big and see yourself as that thin person you know is inside you somewhere yearning to get out. In fact, visualization is a great tool to use toward achieving any goal. When it comes to losing weight, however, you must be realistic. Losing weight takes time and if you set unrealistic or unreachable goals, then all that awaits you is heartache and disappointment.

You must keep your goal in mind all the time so you don't lose sight of it. By doing this, you can make intelligent choices instead of reacting to emotions, stress or other influences. You'll have the opportunity to stay on track.

We've all heard the old saying, "Rome wasn't built in a day." Neither will be your quest to lose weight. It's a long road that isn't going to be quick or effortless. It is the accumulation of the small choices we make along the way that will keep drawing us closer to that future we want to create for ourselves. We have arrived at that final destination when we can say that we've reached our desired weight and now it's time to go on maintenance.

You Are Extremely Valuable

"You are an extremely valuable, worthwhile, significant person, even though your present circumstances may have you feeling otherwise."

~James Newman

So you say you're depressed with being overweight. You're miserable, disheartened, frustrated, restless, angry and wallowing in self pity. You're experiencing trouble staying on your plan for a day, never mind a lifetime. That negative verbiage is echoing, informing you that you're nothing but a fat, disgusting, repulsive, nauseating pig! You couldn't stay on a diet if someone paid you. Maybe even thoughts of suicide have danced there at times.

This negative self-talk needs to be transformed and turned into productive, positive thinking. If anyone deserves success, as well as positive things in their life, it's you. You can have it; it's within your reach. It is never too late to get back on track, even if you've never been on track. You have always struggled with regards to your weight loss program or maintaining a healthy lifestyle and way of eating, but as long as you continue the struggle and don't give up, eventually you'll discover that there are many victories that you have accomplished. It could be something as simple as not gaining weight over a period of time, which is certainly better than the alternative.

You are not alone in your struggle. There are countless numbers of people who've tried a thousand diets and failed a thousand times, and nothing stings more than failure.

In spite of your weight, there is a way out. No matter what road you have traveled, or how many hurdles you have encountered, it doesn't have to lead to defeat unless you let it. YOU have to be the one who says "I've had enough." You are worthwhile even if you experience a setback or two due to whatever situation in your life. Just stay focused and on track and continue the battle another day. Don't mentally wave the white flag of defeat.

What You're Doing Today

"Are you doing what you're doing today because you want to do it, or because it's what you were doing yesterday?"

~Dr. Phil McGraw

Stop blubbering like an infant and take hold of yourself! Feeling sorry for yourself doesn't accomplish anything. Pity parties don't perpetuate success. Do you actually believe that if you keep using the same old methods of losing weight that haven't been affective, that somehow you're going to miraculously attain different results? Be realistic here; if you're not content with your progress thus far, then you must consider an alterative approach to your eating program to get you moving again. You have to do things differently than you are currently doing. Even minor changes in your eating habits can get you moving in the right direction again. Maybe you should consume a little less or start exercising just a little bit more, if you already incorporate exercise in your daily routine.

Ask yourself, "are you doing what you're doing today because you want to do it, or because it's what you were doing yesterday?" If you keep repeating your yesterdays, don't expect to step on that scale and find that it has moved nearer toward your desired weight. It's not going to happen.

What We See

"What we see depends mainly on what we look for."

~John Lubbock

Have you ever walked past a window and seen your reflection? Or walked past a large mirror? Of course you have. But did you ever stop and think about what you saw? If you're not on track with your diet, then you were probably disgusted and loathed the image you saw. Astonished that you could possibly be that enormous and have so much weight to lose, instead of seeing a true representation of where you are today and how far you've actually come. You're afraid to see the real you.

When we're struggling, sometimes those reflections cause us to question our worthiness. We easily become angry and frustrated. Knowing how hard we've worked and yet to see that figure staring back at us is not the form we perceive ourselves to be. Do I really look like that? We ask, doubting everything. How do others see me? I look disgusting, or so says that little inner voice of ours, who is always so anxious to remind us of all our shortcomings.

We must look at ourselves in the present and silence that negative inner voice of ours. We have to reinforce how far we've come and not allow the past to affect us. If we don't grasp the whole picture, then we can't get beyond where we've been.

When this happens, we can't seem to visualize these earlier successes, like changes in clothing size, our new and improved healthy eating habits, or the ability to actually notice a bona fide weight loss. We fail to appreciate all the victories of yesterday at which we have worked so vigorously. We can only seem to set eyes on that reflection in the window or mirror, not noticing how much we have actually changed. We should concentrate on where we started and where we're going and take a harder look at that likeness in the window or mirror, because in all actuality it does point toward our future.

By looking realistically at our entire journey in that window or mirror, instead of only looking at our reflection, it reveals an all-inclusive picture of our future as well. Like a fortune teller's crystal ball, it proves that if we stay diligent and true to our program, we can and will continue to realize results and eventually reach our goals. It can be our inspirational mirror if we let it, offering us hardcore evidence of the path we took yesterday, and today will take us to tomorrow

What We Have to Learn

"What we learn to do, we learn by doing."

~Aristotle

If we keep blaming past circumstances on our being overweight, and our lack of progress to lose it, we overpower our commitment to keep persevering on whatever program we're following. Eventually we will teach our subconscious mind this negative lesson through enough repetition that it will transform into our new belief system.

If we continue communicating damaging and unconstructive thoughts, we are setting ourselves up for certain failure. These thoughts will become our learning, turning any weight loss efforts into nothing but endless, futile attempts of pure hopelessness.

To change our bodies, we must first unlearn our past. If we change our negative thought patterns, our mind-set, the way we think about our eating program or diet, our body image, approach, attitude and what we would like to accomplish, then we can transform and un-learn past failures by learning what to do that will bring us closer to our goals.

What We Anticipate

"What we anticipate seldom occurs; what we least expect generally happens."

~Benjamin Disraeli

Many people confuse the weight shown on their scale as the only measure of the success of their program. Some people weigh daily or several times throughout the day to the point of being obsessed.

There are many ways to "weigh" success: noticing your clothes getting looser or how you have changed unhealthy eating habits into new healthy eating. Being more confident, walking easier, and not running out of breath are just a few of the many other physical and mental changes you should be looking for. These are much more important than worrying about a meaningless number on a scale.

Weight fluctuations are normal throughout the day, as well as daily. Looking forward to stepping on your scale to only see the scale was unchanged may be okay, but if you gained, even if it is ever so slightly, that gain will cause you nothing but disappointment. You will become discouraged and your self-esteem will plummet. It's simply not healthy mentally to get stuck in this sort of "scale paranoia."

So many things influence the scale: water consumption and retention can cause you to go into a tailspin if you don't understand the effects of this on your body, salt intake, sodium in foods, People also tend to forget about the actual weight of the food they eat and women may also retain several pounds of water prior to menstruation. This is very common and the weight will likely disappear as quickly as it arrives. There are many factors that make the scale go up and down, so what we want to happen, with regards to our weight, seldom happens, but if we keep on track and do everything like we're supposed to, when we least expect to see results, they will happen.

We Can't Become

"We cannot become what we need to be by remaining what we are."
~ Max DePree

If you have a goal you want to reach, thinking about it, dreaming about it, hoping or praying about it isn't going to make it happen. You won't get there by doing nothing; it's just not going to happen.

You have to take action; you have to make changes in whatever it is you've been doing that has not helped you reach your goal. At first, if you change one small thing in your daily routine, that will help. Then change another and another until you've changed enough unproductive activities and behaviors into results that will get you where you want to be. After a while they'll add up, bringing you closer and closer to your desired goals.

Simply put, you can't become what you want or get to where you want by remaining the same. You have to make changes or you'll continue to get the same results, which are nothing.

Victory is Won Not in Miles

"Victory is won not in miles but in inches. Win a little now, hold your ground, and later, win a little more."

~Louis L'Amour

When it comes to losing weight and achieving long-lasting results there really is nothing new. We know all about losing weight and almost all programs pretty much have the same basic elements.

When starting on your plan, the best strategy is to take it slow and steady. Don't set yourself up for failure by having unrealistic or unattainable expectations. Remember, there is no quick fix that will help you lose extra pounds and keep them off. You know that in order to lose weight, you must eat fewer calories than your body uses. This is pretty basic stuff that we have learned over the years and from firsthand experience.

Once you start losing weight, don't concern yourself so much with the number of pounds you're losing per week. Pounds lost are pounds not gained and that alone is a victory to be celebrated. You don't have to lose large amounts of weight at one time. When you do lose, keep track either mentally or better yet in a journal of what you ate and did to achieve your results. Then do it again, and later, win a little more by making small changes to what was accomplished and keep right on going.

To Build

"To build may have to be the slow and laborious task of years. To destroy can be the thoughtless act of a single day."

~Winston Churchill

When we put on our weight, it didn't happen overnight, instantaneously, within a week, a month or a year. It took time. So why is it we are so anxious and impatient with ourselves when it comes to losing weight? When losing our excess weight there are no instant solutions. Quick fixes almost always fail, so we must be prepared psychologically for a long haul.

Hundreds of diets, weight loss programs and out-and-out scams promise us quick and easy weight loss. But we can't allow ourselves to fall for that again. By now we should have learned, if through nothing else, but our personal experiences, that they don't exist. There simply are no miracles in weight loss.

Being overweight is not an easy thing to live with or overcome because there are so many complexities to it. There is the physical, the biochemical, and the emotional hurdles to conquer, plus many deep-seated habits to contend with, as well.

Losing weight and keeping it off is going to take time, so we might as well just accept it. It requires effort, exercise, motivation, determination, and an enormous amount of focus to stay on track. It's hard work and can be devastatingly difficult at times.

There will be times that will be filled with celebrated successes, and times where you don't stay on track and you sink to the depths of disappointment, heartache and depression. While it can be wearisome, this is just the way it is.

We need to be diligent, as it takes but a second when our concentration is diverted or interrupted that we can lose sight of our weight–loss goals and go off our program. Then, before we know it, we are vulnerable to an eating frenzy or binge on food we know is not healthy. These actions can carry us far away from our ultimate quest to loss weight.

One thoughtless act against ourselves can destroy us for days or weeks and take us further and further from where we were. It can take everything; our respect, our resolve, our willpower and can make us lose sight of where were going. We have to keep building everyday and recognize that, to reach our mark, it is going to take years. We have to make sure we do not allow one thoughtless act to destroy a single day of our journey.

The World is Full of Suffering

"Although the world is full of suffering, it is also full of the overcoming of it."

~ *Helen Keller*

Have you ever felt that living inside the body of a heavy person is tormenting? It is an anguish that few people understand. In addition to being overweight, we must endure the hurtful way people react to us. People can be so mean: the way they look at us in disgust, make fun of us, whether they are kidding or not, or go out of their way to ignore us. It devastates what little self-esteem we have, and takes our lust for life from us. It sucks all the energy out of us when we have to face the day outside the solitude of our home. We don't like being this way, and hate it as much as the people who taunt us do, maybe more. Society is so judgmental; sometimes we consider it would be better to die than to be so fat.

It is these times when our negative, defeatist side likes to make itself heard the loudest. That negative inner voice of ours that wants to divert us from our aspirations in life and encourages us to eat everything in site. A voice that belittles us and berates everything we've accomplished so far. It makes us question ourselves and our commitment to our diet. It brings us down unlike any living person could ever do to us. Negative thoughts, self-doubt and uncertainty start spinning inside our head, until we are completely overcome with emotion. Then self-pity starts in: we think, poor me, or why me. We look towards the heavens and curse the sky, yelling as tears stream down our cheeks, shouting that no one should have to live like this. No one should suffer this much. Obesity is ruining my life! Can't you just make me normal? We suffer mercilessly. Then the bingeing comes hat can go on for hours, days or weeks.

It is so difficult, that on occasion we just want to declare we're done trying to lose weight and to heck with the consequences. If we allow these destructive negative thoughts to overpower us, however, we are creating a self-filling prophecy that needs to immediately be stopped.

Focus on getting back on your eating program right away, because when it comes to losing weight, you know that staying in control and on track will provide you a better sense of self-worth. You'll feel better about your life, and the way you feel physically and mentally. You know how great it feels to step on that scale and see a loss. We need to hold onto that feeling and make it work for us.

There is no need to suffer from the pain, torment and anguish that we inflict upon ourselves. We can overcome our suffering by sticking to our goal, no matter how time-consuming it may be, until we reach it. By constantly working on our self-esteem, self-confidence, and motivation, in addition to being gentler and kinder to ourselves, we will eventually succeed in achieving our goals.

The Opportunity of Choice

"We are all faced with a series of great opportunities brilliantly disguised as impossible situations."

~Charles R. Swindoll

Choice is the biggest opportunity we have in our lives. When it comes to losing weight and healthy eating, the choices we make will produce the largest impact on the progress we make on our eating plan. There really aren't any "good foods or bad foods." The key is simply moderation and picking the lesser of two evils in the sense that we make an effort to eat the healthier type of the food when presented with choices.

Instead of the fried chicken, pick the grilled. Instead of the fettuccini, pick the fish. Instead of a potato with bacon bits, sour cream, chives smothered in chili topped with cheese, pick a potato with just a little butter. Watch your portions and avoid all-you-can-eat buffets. Have fruit instead of a bag of chips. Substitute a bottle of water for that high calorie sugar packed soda pop, or have a diet soda. It means picking a sensible eating plan, not an unhealthy fad diet.

Take care of yourself. Watch out for words like jumbo, giant, deluxe, biggie-sized or super-sized. Larger portions mean more calories. They also mean more fat, cholesterol and salt. That doesn't mean always eating salads and cottage cheese instead of a hamburger.

It is not always simple to make the appropriate choices. There are plenty of challenges you must deal with, whether it be in a restaurant, convenience store or a vending machine. Be consistent and find ways to follow your plan as much as possible. This healthy approach will make a major difference in your life.

An eating plan or diet doesn't have to be a struggle; it can be, instead, one of life's little pleasures to which we look forward. It doesn't have to be an impossible situation. Constantly elect the healthiest options. Remember the big picture. Be good to your body and take good care of yourself.

The Lust for Comfort

"The lust for comfort, that stealthy thing that enters the house as a guest,
and then becomes a host, and then a master."

~ *Kahlil Gibran*

We all use food for comfort and it certainly can and does seem to make itself right at home. In addition, it masters our emotions and takes control in ways we don't allow anything or anyone else to do in our lives. Sometimes our strongest desire for food as a source of comfort comes when we are emotionally weak or facing a difficult situation, a problem, or are just bored and need something to keep us occupied.

We can learn to control our emotions and not let our emotions sabotage our weight-loss efforts. To do this, we need to recognize the difference between physical and emotional hunger. Somehow, somewhere, we lost our ability to listen and respond appropriately to our hunger signals. In its place we started relying on our emotional cues and fell hostage to them.

If we can distinguish between real hunger and emotional hunger, we can buy a little time to do something other than taking comfort in food. As a result, the sensation to eat will pass. Call a friend, play with your dog, read a good book or watch a movie. Do whatever you need to do to get your mind off eating for a short time.

Whatever you do, avoid getting trapped in an emotional spiral of negative thinking, like nothing really matters, so why care about your weight and eating. When you do this, you are allowing food to master your emotions and setting yourself up for failure.

It's easy to fall into the trap of telling yourself that your reaction to use food as a comfort tool is justified. But we don't have that luxury. Your journey to freedom from eating emotionally and struggling with your weight presents an opportunity for not only a new connection with food, but also a new connection with yourself.

Temptation

"The road to success is dotted with many tempting parking places."

~Author unknown

Temptation is a patient beast. It whispers silently in the wind, diligent, ready to pounce on us at the faintest hint of weakness or disillusionment in our hearts or minds. It waits to lure us away from our diet and steal away the opportunity of us reaching our goals.

There's no question. Temptation is a powerful adversary. If we do not fall prey to it, and just stay level headed, we can uncover the strength to go back to our healthy habits and fight back. Falling prey to temptation is not a time to let go of all the healthy changes we have made. It is a time, instead, to be diligent to our diet.

"Taking it a bite at a time" is a tried and proven method of doing this. It causes us to make the next thing we put in our mouth one that will instantly put us back on track. If we make that next bite of food one that is on our program, in addition to it being a healthy choice, it will keep us from slipping into old negative and destructive eating patterns.

Wellness, permanent life style changes and constant healthy choices is the new face of weight loss. This is what will help us triumph over our weight. We cannot indulge ourselves by parking, we must keep moving toward the goals we desire and the person we outwardly want to become.

Take a Look

"Take a look at those two open hands of yours. They are tools with which to serve, make friends, and reach out for the best in life. Open hands open the way to achievement. Put them to work today."

~ *Wilfred A. Patterson*

It is important to remain open to all that life has to offer, especially when losing weight becomes a challenge, which at times it does.

When dieting becomes difficult and it seems next to impossible to stay on track, this is the point when you must make 'easier said than done' choices to continue achieving a healthy life style and get to your desired weight loss goal.

You have all the tools you need at your disposal: an incredible knowledge by means of trial and error on what it takes to lose weight, the experience of previously losing weight and making the choices that are or aren't in line with your goals, and the ability to gauge where you are and where you're going with your program on a daily basis. You have many significant triumphs that you've completed along your journey thus far to keep you steadfast and on-track. Then there are the friends who support your efforts and who understand your struggle. They are an important tool when it comes to your journey.

You deserve the best in life and when your voyage to lose weight gets a bit grueling, open your hands and use relentless effort. Persevere with your strong sense of commitment to achieve your dreams and your goals, and they will come to pass. Remain enthusiastic and devoted to your healthy eating program, mixed in with a serious amount of determination will result in success. So put them to work for YOU today!

Success

"Success is dependent on effort."

~Sophocles

Nothing happens of its own accord. To achieve weight loss success demands focus, hard work, determination and effort. It is challenging, and it requires commitment. It's not easy, that's for sure. In addition to the effort it takes, we also experience the pressure of the social and emotional fallout of being overweight, which, at times, can be devastating.

Effort is the trials and tribulations we must pay for the added pounds we carry. But we are not alone. One in three American adults is trying to lose weight at any given time, and while their track record for trying is good, their track record for succeeding is not. Too many people get impatient with themselves and don't grant themselves the necessary time it takes to shed their excess weight.

This only leads to heartbreak, disillusionment and frustration. We are too used to this "instant" society of ours of fast food, high-speed cars, microwave meals, while-you-wait photo processing, instant printing, drive-through banking and express lanes.

Today everyone wants immediate and instantaneous results. There are no hard-and-fast rules, however, when it comes to losing weight, except adhering to a weight-loss plan – any plan. As a matter of fact, that is more important than the actual diet regimen itself and that it takes time and effort to be successful.

Strength

"Strength is a matter of the made-up mind."

~John Beecher

When making the effort to lose weight, sometimes it may feel like you're the only person in the world who is on a diet or healthy eating program. Everyone else it seems, is either not watching their weight, or appears to be in total control of their eating and exercise. It's so unfair, especially if you're having trouble with your plan.

Being overweight is a living hell; there are so many negative influences with which we must cope, both physical and psychological. It is a constant battle that we deal with throughout our entire life, even if our weight loss goal is reached and we're on maintenance.

If you're struggling, this is not the time to throw yourself a pity party because life is unfair and you have to struggle. It is not an occasion to allow that negative, self-blaming voice that lives in your head to criticize or to inflict self-hatred upon you. It is, instead, a circumstance when you need to kick your determination into overdrive and implement good judgment. Think about where you've been and the past successes you have had. It is an opportunity to stifle that hateful inner voice.

Give Yourself What You Wish

"Sometimes you just got to give yourself what you wish someone else would give you."

~ Dr. Phil McGraw

How often have you wished or hoped for something to happen, especially when it comes to losing weight? How often have you said it, but not achieved it? You should know by now that wishing to lose weight is never going to happen. So put aside that "wanting and wishing" attitude and get to work.

Nobody wants to be overweight, but, in order to lose weight, you have to give yourself the motivation, determination and fortitude to keep fighting every day until you reach your weight loss goals. You know what needs to be done and how to "just do it." It is hard work, but your success is not based on luck, wishing or wanting. It's based on persistence. If there is anyone who deserves happiness, it is you.

Quit Now

""Quit now, you'll never make it." If you disregard this advice, you'll be halfway there."

~David Zucker

If you're like the average dieter, you have been on and off diets more times than you care to think. One program after another after another, and all you really have accomplished is becoming more and more frustrated and discouraged with yourself and your lack of ability to lose weight and keep it off.

So why not just quit already? When is enough, enough with you? What is it going to take to convince you to throw in the towel and move on? Sure, you'll gain all your weight back. Of course, you'll become increasingly unhappy with yourself as those pounds start creeping back, but the struggle to lose weight will be over.

Just think of all the restaurants and buffets you can go back to and eat to your heart's content without worrying about counting calories or losing weight this week. Think about how you no longer have to go to weekly weight loss meetings. And not caring if you eat a whole bag of cookies or potato chips. Isn't this what you've been longing for, maybe even dreaming about?

Quitting your diet or eating program will be a wonderful feeling; it will be a new-found freedom. This sensation will more than likely not last long, because it will be replaced by something else like self-hate, not to mention your self esteem will go into the toilet, but what the heck! At least you won't have to watch your weight any more. You'll be done with it already. The yoyo dieting, the losing all kinds of weight only to gain it all back over time, will be finished and your obsession with the bathroom scale will be eliminated.

You could quit now, but if you do, you'll never make it. If you disregard this advice, you'll be halfway there. Deep down you know you aren't going to quit. You understand that really isn't what you desire. We may wish we didn't have to watch our food consumption and do all the things it takes to maintain or continue to lose weight, but we know better than that. We understand what will happen to us if we do; we realize the consequences. So we fight another day and don't give quitting one more thought.

Out of Control

"Being out of control is one of the worst feelings in the world, sometimes even worse than pain. It is its own kind of pain."

~Danzae Pace

It's not something that we take pride in, or want to share with, or talk about in the company of others, but we have all done it. Every single one of us has had moments when we are out of control and off our diet or eating program. Sometimes we lose the determination to stick to our goals and binge for a short time. Other times we go for days, weeks and even months until we are able to get back on our plan.

Although we may be filled with regret that we can't un-eat the calories we have consumed, or turn back time, sometimes it is that alone that keeps us off our plan and feeling helpless to stop. Thinking that a setback is cheating and it is not worth the effort because we had a gain only adds to our self-sabotage mindset. An alternative is to make better choices (not perfect, just better) right away. Our weight loss journey is a constant learning curve; you won't get it exactly right every time, but gradually you will.

Mistakes can be our best teachers if we learn from them. We should analyze them carefully without shame. You find yourself in a position where you binged out on something, and I'm fairly confident that you've experienced this one or more times on your weight loss journey. Once it is over, instead of beating yourself up over it, just stop and take a deep breath and think about it.

Think, for instance, about that darned box of cookies you bought for the kids that sat and sat in the cupboard for so long, that it finally called your name loud enough that you just couldn't resist them any longer, so you have one. You feel a little guilty about it, but you're still okay because you are certain that you won't touch the rest. You put them back and think that that is the end of it. Before you know it, those cookies are calling you again, so you have another, promising yourself that the rest are for the kids. Somehow, though, it's you who ends up eating the rest of the cookies and asking yourself what happened.

The answer is not as simple as "I couldn't resist the cookies," or "I had a weak moment." These answers are too raw. Why couldn't you resist the cookies? When did you have a weak moment? Do a complete examination of the cookie episode by going back to the beginning and see where your 'weak moment' started and why it occurred. Were you hungry, tired, angry, depressed? Ask yourself what was happening during the moments before and after you went off your diet or eating plan. Answer the why and you will discover the solution, so maybe there won't be a net time.

Learn from your analysis of the situation. Be aware of everything that led up to the moment and what occurred afterwards. This insight will help prevent future disasters and relapses. Finally, you want to ask yourself, what the moment was like for you when the problem occurred. Were you hungry, or were you tired or angry? What was your emotional state and how did you feel when you went off-track? What snapped you back into awareness to stop your out-of-control behavior? By calmly, but honestly, answering these questions, you'll gain insight and find the answers, as well as their solutions.

Reality

"If you were granted one wish, and only one, what would it be? Of all things . . . Wealth, power, wisdom love, liberty,. . . what would you choose? This may seem fanciful; not so. IT IS REALITY. What you choose to think about, to concentrate on with all your mental power, will, indeed, become a reality. So choose carefully."

~ Thomas D. Willhite

Before you begin any weight loss journey, analyze why you want to lose weight and how you are going to do it to achieve your weight loss goal. That is when the real work begins. Make sure you set realistic goals and get started on an eating plan that will get you to your desired weight loss goal. The next step is to do a mental attitude check in order to understand how our minds and thoughts work.

If you practice positive thinking, you will attract positive results in everything that you undertake in your life, not just your eating plan. If, however, you constantly think how hard it is to lose weight, or that you are always struggling to stay in control, or what difficult roads lay ahead, you will continue to experience difficulty and will be stressed throughout your entire journey. Many people call the use of positive thinking to achieve positive results, the Law of Attraction. The Law of Attraction exists in your life whether you understand or believe it or not.

Basically speaking, on whatever you choose to think and concentrate, that will become your reality. The more positive thoughts that you have about your life and your weight loss plan, the more positive occurrences you will experience in your life and the better the results that you will accomplish.

Start thinking more in terms of what you want from your life and from your eating program than what you don't want. Concentrate on what you want by using self-talk; simply ask yourself "so, what do I want?" In this way, you will end up directing less energy trying to stay on your program and focus more on results that will get you to or closer to your objective.

When you go from thinking about what you don't want to what you do want, you start becoming stronger; you eat right and start seeing more positive end results. It's all part of changing your 'stinking thinking' processes and attracting what you want out of life.

Remember that your thoughts generate either positive or negative consequences. When you use the words "don't, not and no," you exert more energy and focus on what you're thinking. When you change that thinking to what you want, instead of what you don't want, you create changes in your thinking. To stop negative thoughts that will detour you from your goals, picture a stop sign in your mind and yell to yourself to STOP. Then ask yourself, "So what DO I want?" Positive thinking will bring you the goals you desire.

Moving Slowly

"It does not matter how slowly you go, so long as you do not stop."

~ Confucius

Often we find ourselves in the position of feeling depressed because we face such a long journey to reach our weight loss goals. On some days that goal seems so far away, that you doubt if you'll ever reach it. At other times, you can not only see the finish line, but you can taste the sweet victory of success.

The days when that road appears to never end can feel like weeks or months. They feel endless, like looking down a deep well and wondering if there is a bottom to it. You drop in a coin and wait, but you hear nothing. Sometimes that journey can, when you're dieting, literally take months or years to finally accomplish and reach your desired weight. The amount of pounds you need to lose is pretty much in direct proportion to the amount of time it is going to take to lose them. The more weight you have, the longer your road is going to be.

The thing to try and keep in the forefront of your mind is that it doesn't matter how slowly your journey is going. It doesn't matter how long it will take to reach your goal. The more you concentrate on the amount of time it is taking to lose your desired weight, the harder it is going to be to stay focused on reaching your goals and to keep both your level of commitment and determination at their peaks.

It is a tenuous enough road without internalizing additional terms and conditions to make your weight loss journey more difficult. Relax and repeat to yourself that slow and steady is the ideal way to lose weight and keep those pounds off permanently. As long as you do something each day to reach your target, you will feel at peace. You will feel like you are accomplishing something. That feeling of accomplishment will flow over to create many other positive feelings and effects, like having an overall sense of well-being and happiness. Your determination and will seems to be stronger and that there is exhilaration throughout your entire being that you can't really put your finger on, but you feel it.

This experience can make your journey less tiring. While the road ahead may still feel long, it won't be as tedious a road, or seem to be never-ending. Your enthusiasm will carry you. You won't want to stop because you will actually look forward to observing the many changes your body will be undergoing as time goes by, even the small ones. It is those changes and the change in your attitude, in addition to the way you look at your plan and the time it is going to take to reach your goal that will give you a renewed faith and fire in your soul.

Many of us, unfortunately, focus on feeling deprived or tired of the journey, instead of looking at how far they have come. After a while, our diet becomes a burden. It gets boring, so we quit. We can't 'see' that if we just do it another day, fight the fight, win that battle one more time, that we can reach our goal.

You've heard the story many times, as you were growing up about the tortoise and the hare. That 'slow and steady wins the race.' This story has been repeated over the years because there is a moral to it. As long as you don't stop, it doesn't matter how slowly you go.

A New Chance

"Create each day anew."

~Moriehei Ueshiba

Every day is an opportunity to put your past behind you. If you slipped, binged, fell off the wagon or had a back-slide, or whatever you label it, forget about it. Today is brand new with fresh possibilities awaiting you. Yesterday is gone and there is nothing you can do about it, except to move forward and let the mistakes of the past be your teachers of today.

Since today is a new starting point, everything is fresh. Decide to be enthusiastic about your program today. Decide to stay on track. Decide to be determined to stick to your goals for today. Decide to be positive and to recognize how far you have come from where and when you started your weight loss journey.

Let whatever experiences made you detour from your goals yesterday not recur today. Decide if they somehow establish themselves again in your mind that you will look back on them, but only for the lesson in answering why your problem is trying to materialize again. What is happening in this new day, in the now that also occurred yesterday? What experiences are you reliving that are permitting this negative behavior to resurface?

Is it real hunger? Hunger can make us miserable. In fact, hunger is such a powerful feeling that it destroys even the strongest motivation and desire to lose weight. Is it emotions that are steering you off-course, beckoning you to leave all that you've accomplished thus far behind? What is it that wants to take you off the path that will get you where you want to be?

If you are conscious of the what and the why, you have a greater chance to make the correct choices that are healthy for both your program and your mental well-being.

If you start the day off strong, and then something distracts you from stay on course, stop for a moment and simply commit to starting over again from where you are now. Make as many good choices as you can, and commit to improving as the day goes on. Don't dwell on past mistakes or shortcomings. Today is a new day. You should memorize that statement and etch it into your mind. Repeat it to yourself on a regular basis. Understanding the meaning of this statement is what helps turn losers into winners, and failures into successes.

Yesterday's setbacks bring you one step closer to today's successes. The loser of yesterday's race will, with persistence and determination, become the winner of today's race. Any failures you have on your weight loss plan will bring you closer to success. Never give up because of your past. You can correct the things that went wrong yesterday. All of us need to know that every day IS a new day, and every moment is a new chance to grow and make new changes today. So often we think that everything is set in stone. "Today is the first day of the rest of your life." How are you going to choose to live it?

A Long, Long Journey

"If all difficulties were known at the outset of a long journey, most of us would never start out at all."

~Dan Rather

Individuals who have a great deal of weight to lose face an exceptionally long journey to reach their goal. Every moment of every day they struggle to just make it without going off their diet or eating program. They fight to stay in control and not have to start over again. Long Haulers have to gather together enormous amounts of energy, courage, and determination to keep going, in addition to not losing hope or allowing their faith to lapse. It is easy to lose sight of one's objectives or fall prey to negative thinking when there is such a mammoth road ahead. Once you begin letting these destructive thoughts and feelings manifest, they can consume every bit of energy you may have left to fight another day. Before you know it, you're beating yourself up mentally with guilt, followed by a very real physical abuse of your body fro binge eating, stress and depression.

The obstacles Long Haulers face are immense and much harder to overcome than those who have less weight to lose. Most of us would never have started out if we knew what a long, strenuous journey was ahead of us. There are many stumbling blocks to look out for and even more that must be confronted.

Let's face it: those of us who have had of have a great deal of weight to lose do not coexist well with their environment. We face challenges most people can't begin to comprehend.

We are afraid to visit a friend's house because we are terrified at the thought of sitting on a chair or other piece of furniture and having it break. We don't go out to eat because we don't know what type of seating the restaurant has. Not knowing beforehand if we can fit in a booth or if there are tables where we can comfortably sit. Having to repair or buy new things at our own house because our extra weight has caused something to wear or break. Then there are the clothes selections we have; the high prices we pay for what we can get. There are also mirrors and photos, which show us in a less than flattering light. The embarrassment of knowing we let ourselves get to this place in life, the stares, the pity and the resentment we see in peoples' eyes. Then there are also the rude and insulting remarks that are directed our way loud enough to make sure we heard them.

Long Haulers have a more difficult time developing a positive attitude because of self-hate; we despise our self-image; trying to keep in constant control, exerting great effort not to fall off the wagon through will power, in addition to the environmental issues that we face.

There are so many reasons why we overeat as well as why we are overweight. The most important thing to realize is that the habits you have acquired over a lifetime are not going to go away in a couple of weeks. Yet, when we go on a diet, that is what we expect – to become a completely different person in a matter of weeks.

With each turn, you will get to know the road, so it's easier to keep going on the long, long journey. Finally, after a number of stops along the way, a few times where you may have to start all over again, some slow times, and a few wrong turns taking you completely off the path, you will eventually arrive at your destination as long as you never give in or give up.

Face It

"Facing it, always facing it, that's the way to get through. Face it."

~Joseph Conrad

At some point, as hard as it may be, you need to confront reality. You're obese, not fat, pudgy, big boned, overweight, portly, stout, chubby, pleasantly plump, or husky. You are you need to face it, accept it and then get mad as hell and deal with it head on.

We kid ourselves all the time, like when every diet would be "the one" and we usually did not make it. There are many of us who start on a weight loss program (many times over!) thinking, "this is it. This time I am going to do it," only to find that we lose our motivation at the first weigh-in with no weight loss, or heaven forbid, a gain. Why do we do this? Why do we allow a number on a scale to dictate our happiness and level of commitment? Why do we react so harshly and respond with such negative consequences that we affect the progress we made up to that moment. Sometimes we slide further and further away from where we were at that point. For a short time we become numb to the damage we cause ourselves until we snap back to our senses.

It is that "snapping point" when we start a whole new process of behavior. We somehow believe instead of being compassionate and establishing a respectful relationship between food and our program, it is better to feel sorry for ourselves for going off our plan. Then we get angry and start what is sometimes a sadistic process of beating ourselves up.

The punishment is relentless, bordering on emotional torture. We drive ourselves further off our program as resentment, disgust, thoughts of being a failure and that disheartened feeling of being worthless and not deserving of being happy or achieving our goals. There is the sorrow, shame anger and even fear of having to resume our diet once again.

No one knows what it's like to live in a fat body and cope with these feelings, unless you live in a fat body. Nobody knows the anguish better than us. We need to comfort our emotions and not trivialize them. We can't seal ourselves off with cynicism.

We must continue to fight. That is the battle cry you must echo in your mind over and over again when facing the daily difficulty of losing weight and staying on track. Ours is a long, arduous journey littered with failures of every conceivable sort.

Face it, you have to keep going. You have to pick yourself up again. Just don't let a serious or significant setback cause you to lose confidence. Let the knowledge in the fact that you have come this far and have achieved so much to this point be the parachute to keep to keep you from falling. Let it be your own personal bungee cord that will not only "snap" you back to reality, but bounce you right back onto your eating program.

There are no real solutions to our dilemma but patience. The life of a dieter is going to be a series of failures and lots of pick-yourself-up-again sessions. You have to fall in order to rise again. Your concept of yourself has to expand because you are so much more than this disease.

Use awareness to help overcome dieting obstacles that stand in your way. Nothing lasts forever, especially the waves of temptation that lure you away from your goals. Even if they continue, in time the amplitude becomes less and less with longer periods in between until the next instance. There will be a next time, so just "face it."

Change Something You Do

"**You will never change your life until you change something you do daily.**"

~Mike Murdock

A plateau or standstill in your weight loss program can be extremely frustrating, especially if you have been avidly pursuing your plan and were anticipating a loss of some kind. When you know you stayed on track, did what you were supposed to do, sacrificed by not indulging your desires and yet didn't lose weight, it is easy to feel that all that hard work was for basically nothing.

If you continue not losing weight for an extended period of time your frustration levels will rise and your long term commitment levels will plummet to the point you may decide to abandon your program altogether. Your drive, determination and the required ability to stay motivated quickly fades and is promptly replaced by irrational thoughts of "what's the use" and "why bother". It is so disheartening to be diligent and not see some form of movement.

This does not have to be your fate. The "why bother" and "what's the use" list doesn't do much to help us. It only gives us excuses for staying locked in our struggles, often for a lifetime. All we really need to do when we hit a plateau is to stay focused and on our plan, in addition to changing something that we're doing every day. We could lower the amount of calories we eat, take a walk, leave some food on our plate at every meal we eat, drink more water, add more fiber and fruit to our diet. Something different is the key to breaking the cycle that we so desperately need to see.

If we do nothing, then surely we will continue seeing the same results. If we eventually abandon our eating plan of course we will see new results, but they will be in the form of consequences like a weight gain and as much as we may think " why bother" or "what's the use," deep down we know why and aren't really willing to give up on ourselves. So make a change in your daily routine and you'll start to see positive results on the scale again.

When the Problem is Overwhelming

"When the problem is overwhelming and there is not an apparent solution, forget it and move on to more productive thinking. This will give your subconscious a chance to work on the solution."

~Thomas D. Willhite – *Living Synergistically Book*

When you encounter a problem with your eating program like gaining weight or reaching a plateau that you can't seem to get past, you know in your heart you did every thing you could. In fact you have been following it pretty much by the book and you're feeling overwhelmed because you're not seeing the results you desire; then just forget about it.

I know from experience that it is easier said than done because that little inner voice of ours chimes in and starts telling us how appalling we are and that we're not worthy of reaching our goal or ever being happy. We know better than to listen to that unsupportive, critical and often destructive inner voice of ours. It knows how to beat us up and put us down better than any person could ever do. There is no better champion that comes to remind us of our shortcomings and faults than our inner voice.

Instead of giving in and becoming overwhelmed trying to resolve the problem at hand, maybe it is best, when there is no apparent solution to just stop ourselves and forget about it for awhile.

In this way, instead of continuing to beat ourselves up and packing our bags for a pity party, we set the whole situation aside and let our subconscious think about what we have been doing and what actions we can take that will start things moving again in the right direction and get us back on track toward achieving the goals we desire.

This is not only a solution for our eating program but is good for anything we encounter where the problem is overwhelming and there is not an apparent solution.

Avoiding Certain Foods

"Avoid any diet that discourages the use of hot fudge."

~Don Kardong

There are many things you can do that are not healthy for you on a diet. One in particular is deliberately labeling certain foods to eat as good foods or bad foods. Making any food off limits only creates a craving for them because they are forbidden. You actually think of these "off limits" foods more by doing this. The reality is that there are no "bad" foods, just bad eating habits. You can have a scoop of ice cream with a dollop of hot fudge. The key is working it into your food plan and, of course, eating in moderation.

Obviously, there are some foods that are good for you. Carrots, cucumbers, green beans and even broccoli are better for you than candy or ice cream for example. Steamed spinach is better than a slice of white bread, and one of the best vegetables you can eat is a sweet potato. It is loaded with carotenoids, vitamin C, potassium, and fiber.

Dietitians are fond of making statements that all foods can fit into a healthy diet. The main problem is, it is healthy until it is corrupted in the hands of food manufacturers. Once food is process, the unhealthier it becomes. Heavily processed foods are a wonder of today's food industry. The drawback is as food becomes more convenient, there's a price to pay. To assure the "taste" of processed foods, manufacturers add extra sugar, salt and fat, making processed food unhealthier.

Even so, by prohibiting specific foods from your diet or adopting rigid parameters toward a particular food or food groups, you will start thinking about them so much that your cravings for them will soon become totally out of control. Food cravings are complex because it is a combination of motional, chemical and hormonal factors. Usually, triggers like stress, boredom, depression and seeking comfort can lead to cravings. The act of classifying or labeling a food as bad for you and consciously or unconsciously telling yourself you will never eat that food again causes you to yearn for them to the point you can have an episode of uncontrolled bingeing.

This self-delusion of making some foods off limits won't work. We need to reverse food's influences on us and painlessly eat less without depriving ourselves of the foods we enjoy the most.

Moderation is the key ingredient when it comes to consuming those foods that we would normally avoid. A small portion will satisfy your desire for the food in a big way, in addition to bringing you closer to your desired weight-loss goal.

Barriers

"The obstacles you face are . . . mental barriers which can be broken by adopting a more positive approach."

~Jalal ad-Din

Losing weight is a long journey that involves having the endurance to keep motivated for the long haul. This journey is guaranteed to have many barriers that will hinder the best of efforts and intentions. Some will be familiar, taking us by surprise once again. Obstacles we thought we dealt with and overcame appear again before us. Many will be new and unexpected.

Most barriers really aren't as big a hurdle as they may first seem. They can, however, easily send us into a downward spiral that can lead us to feeling defeated, depressed and then we lose confidence in ourselves and our program.

The first thing you have to do is get away from thinking that you can't lose weight. Of course you can! You've done it many times over. It's a matter of strength of mind to keep yourself going one more time until that one more time becomes your last time. For most of us, the reality is if we are having trouble losing and find it difficult to stick to a diet. It means our motivation simply isn't where it should be to lose weight. We need to focus harder on what we want and be realistic about our expectations. If you continue to lose weight only to put it back on again later down the road, then you have to seriously ask yourself what barriers are keeping you from achieving your goals. More likely than not they are not genuine and frankly are excuses you made that are getting in your way.

Maybe it's time to do a reality check and ask yourself why you really eat. What is it that triggers you to go off your eating plan? Have you ever just eaten only to find yourself not too long afterwards opening the refrigerator door? You couldn't be hungry. You just ate! So why are you looking for food? What set your looking for food into motion? Think back to what you were doing before the urge hit you to go foraging for food. Think logically and clearly; the answers are right there in your head. Ask yourself what influenced you to take this course of action. Even if you can't discover the cause, believe in your ability and mental capacity to break through the barriers that present themselves.

Don't expect a quick fix. If you have a lot of weight to lose, it will take time to reach your goal. On a healthy diet program, you generally will lose two to three pounds per week. Sure we all wish for a faster, accelerated diet program. We often think it's not worth the effort or claim that we have no support network to help us over the many hurdles that act as barriers.

The right mindset, positive thinking accepting responsibility for your actions and the consequences of what you eat will move you from someone who says they can't lose weight to someone who can. Just starting a diet is not going to get you to your goal because there are so many barriers ahead. It takes work and a daily commitment to help you through the rough spots.

You know how to lose weight. You know that if you consume fewer calories and exercise you will see results. That is the common ingredient of all diet and healthy eating programs. Clinical studies have proven that the most important factor to overcoming weight-loss obstacles, barriers and achieving success is attitude. You may not believe all this, but the fact is that the desire may be in your heart to succeed, but you need to put it into your head. What you think affects how you feel about your program and your self-worth. This translates into the type of action you take to get you where you want.

Perseverance

"When the world says "Give up," Hope whispers, " Try it one more time."

~Author unknown

Perseverance is commitment, hard work, determination, patience and staying power. It is being able to tolerate the tough and difficult times calmly. It is trying again and again, especially for something at which you weren't successful the first time around.

Losing weight tests your perseverance. It establishes how seriously you're committed to your program. It will push you to the breaking point or catapult you to victory.

Perseverance will force you to try again when something doesn't work for you. It will compel you to finish your weight loss journey, come hell or high water. It will demonstrate that you have what it takes, not to give up on yourself and keep striving no matter how difficult the day may be or what lies ahead of you.

Perseverance will make you face and accept your circumstances. It will make you take a good look at what you're made of, who you are, and dive deeper into your mind and examine your feelings. It will eventually make you healthier allowing you to take better care of yourself. Perseverance will make you learn and grow from your successes and failures.

When you stop forging ahead because you are in such despair, and just don't feel that you can go on, it is perseverance that makes you take that one more step you need to keep going.

You need to establish a 'lifers' mentality when it comes to losing weight. 'Lifers' is a military term for people who are committed to something for the long haul. A lifer has a very different mindset than most of us. They realize that there might be obstacles to overcome, but they decide in advance that they will go through them, around them, or over them, but they do not allow those hindrances to stop them. It may take some doing and might even include support from other, but in the end their undertaking gets accomplished. Are you a lifer? Could you be? Do you have what it takes to persevere no matter what is thrown in front of you?

True perseverance is an attitude of the heart. It helps you through the tough times. It helps you when you want to quit. It keeps you going for that long journey ahead of you, through the struggle and emotional roller coaster rides.

It won't be easy; no one can count your calories, keep you from overeating, indulging, bingeing, or exercising. It's your internal self-motivation, discipline and self-determination and it's all up to you. As long as you keep moving forward, no matter what gets in your way, you will reach your goal.

If you believe that weight loss is easy and quick, you are denying the well-known truth that losing weight is not quick and easy. Weight loss and healthy living are two factors that do, however, go hand in hand and don't contradict each other. The body prefers small and slow changes rather than sudden transformations. With reasonable goals and expectations, you are not going to obtain the desired results overnight. A healthy weight loss program, moderate exercise, determination and the magic of perseverance in time, you will achiever the healthy body and appearance you have always wanted.

Disappointed Passion

"It is foolish to pretend that one is fully recovered from a disappointed passion. Such wounds always leave a scar."

~Henry Wadsworth Longfellow

Why is it that other people's evaluations of your weight loss are so much more important that your own? Especially from the same people who were unkind towards you about your weight in the beginning. Why does it matter?

Why is it when we receive compliments about our weight loss, we are pleased and internally grateful that someone noticed? More importantly, why is it that people don't notice our hard work and diligence? When this happens, our old eating habits see to slowly creep back eventually overtaking the new healthier ones.

It's as if you had to hear accolades from someone to stay the course, and without that acknowledgment of you weight loss, you have given yourself permission to gain your weight back. Break out of the disappointment and hang in there! This is for you, not for other people. Besides, your friends might be holding back to save you from feeling embarrassed and humiliated in the event you regain the weight. If they give you a lot of praise and then next time they see you and you had gained you weight all back, what are they to say?

It is disappointing that your friends or family members don't notice or acknowledge your hard work. We, however, are supposed to do it for ourselves. It is, of course, totally understandable to want the support and encouragement and attention of those who are close to us, but it truly doesn't matter what others think or notice. If you recognize not to expect compliments of comment of any kind about your weight you won't be let down.

The path you take on your weight loss journey can be a lonely one. Those who love you will support you, encourage you and be there for you, but you must be there for yourself with the same vigor and excitement that you want from others about your accomplishments. Disappointment comes from within as does confidence, determination, fortitude, endurance and the guts to continue fighting for what you want.

There is nothing in this world that someone else can give you that you can't give to yourself. If the world does not take notice right away keep doing whatever it takes to bring you closer to your desired goal. One day, then, when you least expect it, you'll be surprised because people will observe the changes you have made to yourself physically and mentally.

People, in general, are too focused on themselves to notice other people's accomplishments. It doesn't necessarily make them awful people or awful friends, it's just human nature. So never mind other people's obvious oversights! What's important is that YOU know you lost weight and you know what you accomplished and you're healthier because of it. Your friends may not be complimenting you, but your body is thanking you each and every day.

Reward Yourself

"The highest reward for a man's toil is not what he gets for it but what he becomes by it."

~John Ruskin

You shouldn't take dieting so seriously. Sure, it's a serious business, but that doesn't mean that a diet has to be so serious that it becomes stressful. A diet isn't the end of the world; it's a beginning. Find joy in your new-found journey. Look for changes in your thinking, attitude, and appearance. Smile at the little things like clothes fitting loose. Whatever you do, don't let the scale be your only guide. Laugh a little, stop and smell the roses. Bask in your successes along the way.

Take action every day that will lead you closer to your goal. You don't have to make drastic changes, just small ones. Add to them a little at a time. Before you realize it, these small additions will add up to noticeable accomplishments. So much so, that friends and family will send comments and kudos your way. They will be sincerely happy that you are losing weight and will share in your triumph.

Since a lot of people who are heavy are givers, it may be hard to accept these pats on the back, but enjoy them and allow them to lead you further. Take each compliment to heart and take pleasure in them. Start rediscovering life and live each day to its fullest. Reward yourself by doing things you like and that bring you pleasure.

Don't be so pessimistic; start being kinder to yourself and look for the slightest advancements. Acknowledge each and every one of them as you lose weight. In this way, you're telling yourself that you're actually doing it this time. Buy yourself something that makes you feel good. If you keep a weight loss journal, write down not only your loss, but what kind of reward that you gave yourself. Whatever you do, don't use food as a reward; make it something you want for yourself like a CD, makeup, or a new piece of clothing. Break out of your comfort zone and do things you normally wouldn't do.

This is important because when you have a great deal of weight to lose and are not close to your desired weight, the road ahead seems to be endless and in many cases feels like you will never get to the weight you desire. The whole process can make you feel hopeless. Whatever you do, don't look at a weight loss program as a punishment for letting yourself get fat. Stop yourself from thinking negatively. Don't say, "Because I ate everything I wanted before, I deserve to suffer now." This mindset is not mentally healthy.

Set up lots of short term objectives that collectively bring you to your long-term weight loss goal. A short-term reachable goal could be drinking more water each day than you are currently doing. Clearly visualize that in your mind. Be very specific with your goals. Don't just say, "I need to drink more water." Say, "I will drink two more glasses of water a day than I normally do." Or if six glasses of water is normal for you, and you want to drink two more glasses of water a day, say, "I will drink eight glasses of water each day." When you start to actually do this, make a point to do something for yourself as a reward. Make your reward unique to you and remember that your reward doesn't have to break the bank. Your reward should be something that will motivate and excite you at the same time.

The Holidays

"Holiday or no, the world goes on."

~James Michael Ullman

The holidays are not an excuse to give up on your diet or temporarily set it aside. It is a time of year when you need to be realistic about your program and strive to maintain your weight. Unfortunately, for those of us with a weight problem, many holidays revolve around food. As a result people gain weight during these times. This could be from the foods that surround us, or from emotions that are invoked during these times.

You know it's coming, whether it is the "Four of July, Easter, Christmas, Chanukah, or Memorial Day. You need to recognize in advance that there are going to be challenges ahead of you with which you don't normally have to contend. Many people find that the temptations of the holidays are too much for them, and simply give up on healthy eating. If, however, you recognize that there will be challenges over the holidays, prepare for them. It needn't be a total surrender of everything that you worked so hard to achieve.

The most important thing to have during any holiday is an advance strategy. If you arm yourself ahead of time you will be able to get through the holiday unscathed. Instead of dwelling on the fact that you have to limit your eating or avoid all kinds of foods because you're on a diet, try changing your thinking. Adjust your inner voice and the messages that you send yourself from thoughts of being deprived or limited, to one of a person who isn't trying to lose weight.

Think of all the positive advancements you have made so far and remind yourself that you want to continue eating healthy foods. If you think about healthy eating instead of avoiding all those wonderful foods, then you will find that you can eat a nice variety of things and still keep on track.

Teach you inner voice defensive thinking, so when temptations are in front of you , there are options that are preset in your mind that will protect you from straying too far off your weight loss program. Don't think of restrictions and don't try losing weight during the holidays; just focus on maintaining your weight and not gaining. That will be challenging enough for you.

Enjoy your time with friends and family. Food is certainly a large part of many holidays, but it isn't the main focus. Concentrate on celebrating being reunited with people you haven't seen in a while. Create new and lasting memories with those people. Remember to eat in moderation and just relax a little. It's okay once in a while to eat too much, but also remember it is okay to take smaller servings. Have refill later and, by all means, it is okay to say "No" to food that is offered. Most of all, have fun.

Keep your inner voice actively working for you during these trying times for dieters. Remind yourself occasionally that a holiday is not an opportunity for overzealous eating or bingeing. Perspective is important: if you do overeat on one day, that isn't going to break your program. You may not even gain weight because it usually takes more than one day of overeating to cause a weight gain. Whatever you do during a holiday, return to your healthy eating plan the very next day and get back on track without guilt or beating yourself up.

Sick of It

"I wish I had an answer to that because I'm tired of answering that question."

~Yogi Berra

Losing weight requires a lifestyle change and a commitment to a long and, in most cases, an endless course of action. We don't need advice nor do we need to be convinced by anyone of the why's or how's to lose weight. We don't need friends or family, as well-intentioned as they may be, asking us questions about our weight or politely trying to prod us into action.

The only people who can do this is us. We are the ones who have to change what we do and how we think so we can get started and take even the smallest of steps toward our weight loss goals. We know it is all a matter of choices, even the one that put our weight on in the first place. Being overweight, we know what it takes to diet and to be successful at it, maybe not to the point where we lose all our unwanted weight and keep it off, but if anything else, we do know how to drop pounds once we put our minds to it.

When we do commit to an eating plan or program and stick to it, we lose weight. It's all rather simple: fewer calories in, more pounds off. We've done it hundred of times. So how do we do it differently this time in order to stop the cycle of losing and gaining? Can it be done, or are we destined to 'roller coaster' our entire lives?

Those of us who do lose weight, ninety to ninety-five percent don't keep it off in the long term. That is extremely discouraging, but there are plenty of people who do lose weight and keep it off permanently. So maybe we should learn what they do before we are staring maintenance in the face. If we apply to ourselves what other people do to keep their weight off, then we, in turn, should be able to keep off the pounds we lost so far, and yet continue to lose.

Maintainers, as I call them, do several things that most of us on our weight loss journey don't, although we're more than aware of these things and should be doing them. Most people who have lost their weight and have kept if off for a year or more, eat breakfast every morning. That really isn't news to us; we've heard this hundreds of times over how we should not skip meals.

In addition to following a healthy eating program, most long term maintainers regularly exercise and track their activities. They weigh themselves daily, although I am not an advocate of weighing yourself all the time. If this is what it takes to lose weight and keep it off, so be it. They keep precise food journals and meticulously watch for changes by self-monitoring everything.

Why not us too? We all should follow 'maintainers' examples and do the same things they do every day. It will keep us not only continuing our weight loss journey, but also be successful at not gaining back any of the weight we lost while on it. We can learn from them, emulate them and maybe break that chain of 'roller coasting.'

We all wish we could find that Holy Grail of answers to our weight loss. Until then, by combining the techniques and methodologies of those who have gone before us, and who have succeeded, we can eventually become not only our own example of achievement, but someone else's as well.

Eating When You're Hungry

"The obstacles you face are . . . mental barriers which can be broken by adopting a more positive approach."

~Jalal ad-Din

You would think this would be obvious. After all, it makes total sense. "Eat when you're hungry," and "Don't eat when you're not," but for some reason we rarely heed that adv ice as prudent as it may be.

Many people who are on weight loss programs have difficulty disseminating the difference between real hunger and emotional "feel good" hunger. Often we don't even know what it is like to feel full and to know when enough food is enough, never mind what type of hunger they are experiencing.

You need to get in touch with your body and start using food as fuel instead of a temporary crutch to satisfy some emotions with comfort food. This entails being aware of your body's needs and not eating if we're not hungry. With people who are overweight as we all know too well, this normally happens to us when some emotional reaction to something triggers us and we want to eat something, anything.

The best way to become aware of which type of hunger you're experiencing is to track it. Keep a diary or food log, writing down what you eat, when you ate it, and what you're feeling at the time. Eventually a pattern will emerge and you will actually be able to "see" this negative behavior of using food as a comfort. If nothing else, over time it will become much clearer to you. It is going to take effort to do this until you start to see it, so perseverance is important, but, hey, if anyone is worth it, you are! After a while of doing this, you will actually unconsciously ask yourself if you're really hungry or not. Best of all, by paying attention to your hunger, you'll find the answer to your question. As a result, you'll be able to make the necessary choices to keep you on track and moving forward. This will also keep you from eating until you are stuffed out of your gourd.

So the next time you're hungry, take a moment and ask yourself a few questions, slow down while you're eating, and stop every now and then to consciously check your fullness level. This will help you to help yourself by gaining control over your eating. Many people eat when they feel upset, angry, sad, lonely or fearful. Emotions such at these can be powerful triggers and will detour you from your goals.

With constant practice, however, you'll become sensitive to knowing when you're full. Of course, making healthy choices and eating well helps promote a positive mental attitude, as well as better physical health.

Will Power

"It's not that some people have willpower and some don't. It's that some people are ready to change and others are not."

~James Gordon

When talking about having the willpower to diet – willpower is nothing more than the ability to control a self-destructive impulse. It is the capability to overcome the desire to indulge in unnecessary bad habits and find the inner strength to triumph over it. You need willpower so you can have power over your thoughts before they lead to an unwelcome action like bingeing. The more control you have over your thoughts, the stronger this ability will become. Once you become the master of your own mind, you will enjoy inner peace and feel better about your diet or healthy eating program.

Willpower is really nothing more than commitment. You have to make a commitment to yourself to stay on your program and have strategies in place if your commitment falters. Many people think those of us who are overweight lack willpower, but this is not true. Although when our diet fails, the lack of willpower is one of the first things to which we will point. Diets fail because of lack of desire, not willpower.

The truth is that we weren't committed enough. We didn't desire it bad enough to do whatever it takes to reach our goal. We allowed ourselves the indulgence of going off our plan and satisfying some temporary desire instead of stopping for a moment and working through it. It is your desire that will keep you going for the long haul, not willpower. Willpower and the ability to use it to stick to a weight loss diet or program has nothing to do with will – and everything to do with changing your attitude towards your commitment and how you think about food.

Not to pop your bubble, but lately, much of the scientific community has dispelled the importance of willpower in weight loss. While sheer willpower can work in some cases, it usually doesn't work in the long term. It is our commitment that has to be strong, not our willpower to overcome a moment of temptation. The notion of not having enough willpower to stick to a diet is self-defeating. It's another excuse to make it okay, or to justify going off our plan. Well, it's a lie and it isn't okay. We need to stop blaming outside influences and start pointing the finger where it belongs and that is at our own commitment levels. We need to take responsibility for our actions or lack or them and stop putting so much value on willpower. While this may seem like you're using willpower to overcome the desire to eat a certain food, what you're really experiencing is an unconscious or, in some cases, a conscious decision to stay committed.

Commitment requires you to change the way you are currently approaching your diet and replace it with a healthy eating plan. Make the right choices in the types of foods we eat. When you make the right choices and resist foods that you know are not healthy, this is your commitment talking to you. It's showing you that you have it in you to decide , and the power to go down the right path that will take you where you want to be on your eating plan.

Willpower is the dieter's nemesis. If you don't have it, you use it as the reason you can't stick to your diet. If you do have it, you never have enough of it because it doesn't last. So when it comes to weight loss you need more than willpower – you need commitment.

There isn't Enough Time

"Don't say you don't have enough time. You have exactly the same number of hours per day that were given to Helen Keller, Pasteur, Michelangelo, Mother Teresa, Leonardo da Vinci, Thomas Jefferson, and Albert Einstein."

~H. Jackson Brown, Jr.

How often have you said you don't have enough time to diet properly? "I'd take the time to prepare healthy meals, but I just don't have the time." For many of us, our time is stretched thin and it is hard to find the time to prepare healthy meals, right?

You know what? "There isn't enough time" is an excuse and we certainly know how to milk it for everything it's worth when it comes to losing weight. Because of this one excuse, we actually stop ourselves from sticking to a healthy routine, gain weight and face heartache, disappointment and have to struggle more than we should. It's downright lame.

You need to stop making excuses to justify the fact that you're struggling to lose weight. The no time excuse can seem valid to us, especially with the busy lives most of us lead today. It is up to you, however, to decide how important losing weight is to you. If it is important to you, then you need to learn to put yourself first.

Putting yourself first is something many people with weight problems aren't used to doing. If you're like most people with a weight problem you are most likely a "giver" and not accustomed to putting yourself first. The way you think about yourself will affect how you will succeed with your weight loss program. The more excuses you make, the more you will fail. So your losing weight is for the most part a mental or emotional issue.

You know what to eat. You know how much food to consume. You know about calories, fat content and everything else there is to dieting and you know that you must participate in some form of physical exercise. The next step is to overcome weight loss excuses. To do that, first you need to understand the reason you're making them and why you feel the excuse is legitimate.

Do you really have no time at all to prepare healthy meals? No time at all? Come on, you know you have some time even if life is hectic if it was really important to you. It just takes commitment and perseverance and how you go about your daily routine. You need to make changes to accommodate what you need to do to make yourself a success on your eating plan. As ridiculous as it may sound, if you're so consumed with everyday life, you can't make the time for you then maybe a diet or healthy eating plan isn't right for you just now. Maybe you should give up and set your weight loss plans aside.

I say ridiculous because if you want it bad enough you can make anything work and anything happen. You just need to rethink the way you do certain things and do them a little differently. Discipline yourself; make the time, after all it's there. You know it is but it is easy to use time as your scapegoat.

If you're committed, in time you will find your lifestyle changes aren't as burdensome as you first thought they would be. Finding the time for yourself will be easier than you thought, especially when you start seeing and experiencing results from your efforts.

How are you going to move forward losing weight if you keep telling yourself that you don't have enough time to do it properly? You can't, that's how. So don't put off you weight loss program another day. No more excuses! There's no room for them and there is no time like the present – no ifs and or buts about it.

Overeating

"More people commit suicide with a fork than with a gun."

~Author unknown

Have you ever noticed that your hand or mind moves toward food when you aren't even hungry? It happens to all of us now and then. I'm not talking about being a compulsive overeater. I'm talking about how you're doing great on your weigh loss plan or diet and all of a sudden, POW! You're bingeing.

We can't end our relationship with food because we need food to fuel our body. It would be nice if we didn't ever have to eat again and not worry about food but that is not our reality. So we have to make changes about how we think of food. We need to become balanced in our eating and stop continuously depriving ourselves of various foods to the point that they constantly call our name or we think about them so much that we crave them.

If you desire a particular food, have it. Just set boundaries in advance. If you have one cookie, that doesn't mean you may eat the whole box. Some people, of course, can't eat just one. For them, this may be bad advice. It may be better to have something that isn't readily accessible to you, such as something you truly savor from your favorite bakery, one you don't go to very often.

Our relationship with food doesn't have to be all or nothing. We don't have to overdo it either. If you take a moment to look at what you have on your plate in front of you, there is an instance in time when you can ask yourself if this is really what you want to eat. It gives you time to think of what you're about to consume. Is there some mindless act of piling on food that was almost robotic-like? Or is this food what you really want? More often than not, if you really think about it before you put that first bite into your mouth, you'll clearly see that your selections are not going to get you to your goals, and weren't the wisest choices you could have made.

If you still can't stop yourself from overeating, start off taking small bites of the food you chose. Take your time with your meal and enjoy each bite. Sometimes this is enough to bring us to our senses and stop our destructive behavior.

Also don't be a diet buster. When you're done, you don't have to save the leftovers. You don't have to not waste food or save it for hungry kids overseas. Throw it away or make up you mind it isn't some unwritten law that you have to finish it or can't share it with someone. It's not your job to make it all gone.

You are ultimately in control of your eating and your relationship with food no matter what. It's just food; it's not going to solve your problems. While it may temporarily make you feel better, once you realize you've fallen off the wagon you're going to be miserable. You will feel regret, guilt and even shame.

Ask yourself how important is the food you're about to eat? How important is your weight loss goal? It just takes a few seconds to stop overeating. Is your weight loss REALLY important to you? Is it kind of important to you, or is it just a passing thought? It helps to get specific with your goals because this will always keep you on track.

Most of all, ask yourself if you are really hungry right now. As babies, we were born knowing to eat when we were hungry, and to stop when we were full. As we got older, however, we used food differently and unlearned that instinct we had as babies. We need to find that balance again and relearn to eat when we are hungry and stop eating when we are full without overeating – this is probably one of the main keys to healthy eating and living.

Depression, Stress and Weight Gain

"A lot of what passes for depression these days is nothing more than a body saying that it needs work."

~Geoffrey Norman

Did you know that depression and weight gain often go hand in hand? Who would have guessed? Like we don't know the answer to that one! Not everyone knows this, but one of the main reasons for this besides our uncanny ability to blame ourselves for every stumble we encounter along our weight loss journey is the chemical, Serotonin. Serotonin is the chemical that helps us to stay content. Why do you think we love carbohydrates so much? That's because carbs help increase our Serotonin levels. It figures, doesn't it?

In addition many of us who fail miserably at losing weight and who are vulnerable to depression and weight gain could be the result of eating too much carbohydrate-rich foods. So on top of everything else we have to contend with, we have this factor as well.

Just remember: losing weight is not a race. It's a journey and often a long one. If you have a bad day or a bad few days it doesn't mean that you have to throw in the towel and give up. It doesn't mean that you have to sink into a state of deep depression. There is always tomorrow. Too many dieters think that if they worked hard all week only to show no weight loss or even a slight gain, they might as well just give up.

Giving up on your diet, means you're really giving up on yourself. People who are successful on a weight loss program understand that the road to their goal has many pot holes. There are lots of bad days; it's the law of dieting nature. That doesn't mean that you give in to it or give up. It means you fight that much harder and stay true to yourself and your weight loss plan. This way, instead of sinking into a depression, you will actually experience a sort of at ease feeling within yourself and not become stresses. That's a good thing because stress in and of itself causes depression and weight gain.

Some experts say that depression contributes to weight gain. Others say being overweight leads to depression. Either way the two are definitely connected. Eventually you get caught in a terrible, vicious cycle that keeps repeating itself over and over again. You eat, you gain weight, and you become depressed. The more weight you gain the worse you feel about yourself. This includes feelings of hopelessness, low self-esteem and low self-worth.

Eating healthy and sticking to our predetermined eating plan or diet is difficult to do if we're stressed, because stress, more often than not, is followed by feeling depressed. Although being stressed doesn't automatically make you gain weight, it is more difficult to maintain healthy eating habits. Many of us eat more to find comfort, to make an attempt to fulfill some sort of emotional needs during stressful times. This makes you gain weight. Also, it is important to understand if you're taking any type of medication for anxiety that could cause you to gain weight.

So while the subject is actually pretty heavy, lighten up on yourself a little and keep focused on following your dream of losing weight. Keep you goal in mind and be in the present, instead of focusing so much on the future. Whatever you do, don't dwell on the past. You can't change it, so let it go. Your "Perception is reality," so perceive to believe and you can get where you want to be. Just take it slow; this way there is no stress, which can lead to depression, which will lead to . . . you guessed it . . . weight gain.

RESOURCES

The following resources are for informational and convenience purposes only, and in no way constitute and endorsement, expressed or implied, unless noted by an "*" by the author. Under no circumstances has any compensation been made to the author by any parties.

*WEIGHT LOSS SUPPORT GROUPS

T.O.P.S. – (Take Off Pounds Sensibly)
Website: www.tops.org

This is the program that keeps me on track and accountable – Morris Katzoff - T.O.P.S. is a non-profit, noncommercial weight-loss support group. Since 1948, T.O.P.S. has provided its members with weekly meetings that include positive motivation and reinforcement, along with tips on healthy food choices. T.O.P.S. promotes learning from each other by sharing real-life situations and, together, finding strategies to manage or overcome obstacles that may stand in the way of losing weight. Weekly meetings incorporate private weigh-ins to keep participants accountable, as well as encourage weight loss through recognition and rewards.

Overeaters Anonymous
Website: www.oa.org

Overeaters Anonymous offers a program of recovery form compulsive overeating using the twelve steps and twelve traditions of OA. Worldwide meetings and other tools provide a fellowship of experience, strength and hope, where members respect one another's anonymity. OA charges no dues or fees. It is self-supporting through member contributions. Unlike other organizations, OA is not just about weight loss, obesity or diets; it addresses physical, emotional and spiritual well-being. It is not a religious organization and does not promote any particular diet. To address weight loss, OA encourages member to develop a food plan with a health care professional and a sponsor.

WEIGHT LOSS PLANS

The Carbohydrate Addict's Diet
Website: www.carbohydrateaddicts. com

This is a program that in all essence saved my life – Morris Katzoff – The Carbohydrate Addicts Diet (CAD) – The Carbohydrate Addicts' Lifespan Program (CALP) from Doctors Richard and Rachelle Heller. Through their tireless research and dedication, the Doctors Heller offer a step-by-step, results-oriented solution to permanent weight-loss. Their program shows how carbohydrates contribute to cravings and weight gain. If you are carbohydrate addicted, this book will give you vital information, in addition to plenty of delicious, easy to prepare recipes to keep insulin levels in check and the ammunition to totally eliminate carbohydrate addition and craving forever.

Weight Watchers
Website: www.weightwatchers.com

Weight Watchers is one of the most popular weight-loss plans among dieters. Weekly meetings off Weight Watchers' customers guidance to help them succeed on their weight-loss journey, as well as support, learning behavior modification, tips on healthy eating habits, exercise, healthier eating habits and making smarter food choices. Weight Watchers is a support environment emphasizing exercise, an eating plan that allows participants to eat what they like, nutritional advice on staying satisfied and losing weight at a healthy rate and over time gaining the knowledge to keep it off.

RECOMMENDED READING
To help transform your negative, self-destructive thinking

Your Erroneous Zones, by Doctor Wayne W. Dyer

Doctor Wayne W. Dyer explains our self-sabotaging behavior and what we can do about it. If we can take charge of our lives, we can change our way of thinking and get rid of negatives such as guilt, procrastination, and boredom.

Pulling Your Own Strings, by Doctor Wayne W. Dyer

Pulling Your Own Strings offers positive and practical advice for learning how to pull your own strings and live your life on your own terms. Dyer delivers dynamic techniques for dealing with other people and avoiding victimization.

The Secret, by Rhonda Byrne

Supporters of this New Age self-help book on the Law of Attraction hail *The Secret* as a groundbreaking and life-changing work, finding validation in its thesis that one's positive thoughts are powerful magnets that attract wealth, health, and happiness. *The Secret* is motivational book with an abundance of "you-can-do-it" encouragement on positive thought for positive results. In addition, you will learn how to have, do or be anything that you desire.

OTHER BOOKS

The Carbohydrate Addict's Lifespan Program: a Personalized Plan for Becoming Slim, Fit and Healthy in Your 40's, 50's 60's and Beyond, by Dr. Rachael F. Heller and Dr. Richard F. Heller

From the #1 "New York Times" bestselling authors of the *Carbohydrate Addict's Diet*, Doctor Rachael F. Heller and Doctor Richard F. Heller. The authors assert that consuming too many carbohydrates causes the body to increase insulin production and that excessive amounts of insulin prevent weight loss. This version of their plan targets common weight-loss issues of middle-aged people and provides a two-week program that may eliminate carbohydrate craving and hunger pangs.

HEALTH AND NUTRITION

American Diabetes Association
Website: www.diabetes.org

Founded in 1940, the American Diabetes Association is the nation's foremost authority on diabetes research, information and advocacy on all diabetes-related issues. Their mission is to prevent and cure diabetes and to improve the lives of all people who are affected by diabetes.

NAACO – The Obesity Society
Website: www.obesity.org

A scientific society dedicated to the study of obesity. Since 1982, The Obesity Society has been committed to encouraging research on the causes and treatment of obesity, and to keeping the medical community and public informed of new advances.

American Dietetic Association
Website: www.eatright.org

The American Dietetic Association (ADA) is the largest organization of food and nutrition professionals. They serve the public by promoting optimal nutrition, health and wee-being. ADA members are the nation's food and nutrition experts, translating the science of nutrition into practical solutions for healthy living.

WebMD
Website: www.webmd.com

WebMd is the nation's leading source for information on health and wellness on the internet.

PERSONAL AND BUSINESS RELATIONSHIP BUILDING TOOLS

Send Out Cards
Website: www.247cardshop.com

From the convenience of your computer, you can select from one of over 10,000 stock cards or create your own custom designed card with pictures inside or out. Your imagination is your only limitation. You can then write a message (in your own handwriting with your own signature) and with the click of your mouse, send a store-bought quality printed greeting card or post card. **SendOutCards will print it, stuff it in a real envelope, stamp it and send it in the mail for you.** It's fast, easy and fund. And a reminder system will even tell you when a card is needed, ALL FOR RIGHT AROUND $1.00 with postage.

A Word of Thanks

Thank you for purchasing this book. I sincerely hope it will be of value to you and that it will continue to be a source of encouragement, inspiration and motivation on your weight loss journey.

Morris C. Katzoff
P.O. Box 86187
Phoenix, AZ 85080
Office – (623) 582-2600
Fax – (775) 924-8245
Email – morris@morriskatzoff.com
Website – www.morriskatzoff.com